Days Like These

The upside and backside of cancer

SUE TREDGET

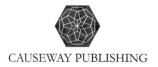

CAUSEWAY PUBLISHING

Published in Western Australia by
Causeway Publishing
Wembley Downs, WA 6019
www.suetredget.com

First published in Australia 2023
Copyright © Sue Tredget 2023

 A catalogue record for this
book is available from the
National Library of Australia

Creator: Sue Tredget
Title: Days Like These
ISBN: 978-0-6458392-0-3
ISBN: 978-0-6458392-1-0 (ebook)

Cover design and layout: Rhianna King
(www.rhiannaking.com.au)

Disclaimer
All care has been taken in the preparation of the
information herein, but no responsibility can be accepted
by the publisher or author for any damages resulting from
the misinterpretation of this work. All contact details given
in this book were current at the time of publication, but are
subject to change.

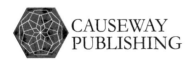

For Marita, who makes everything brighter.

Contents

SUE TREDGET

Overture

There are days when you finally make an appointment to see your GP about something that's been niggling you, something that doesn't feel quite right, something you think is nothing. And he takes one look at that something and everything starts to spiral.

There are days when you have scans and biopsies and surgery and needles in your arm and blood sucked from your body and fluids injected through your veins and instruments probing multiple orifices.

There are days when you lie under blinding lights, your life in the hands of total strangers as your world continues to spin out of control. There are endless days that turn into weeks, that turn into months of treatment that challenges your strength and tests your spirit every minute of every day.

There are days when you look in the mirror and no longer recognise yourself.

And then there are those ordinary days when your world isn't spiraling or upside down and back to front but everyone and everything grates.

When the driver in front of you hogs the right-hand lane while maintaining an infuriating speed precisely 3km/h below the limit.

When the frosty receptionist tells you with no small amount of glee that there are absolutely no free appointments for the next three months.

When that acquaintance who thinks she's so much more important than you takes great delight in highlighting her own wonderfulness and your shortcomings. When that co-worker takes credit for your ideas.

When the tradesman who promised you faithfully your job would be completed by the weekend decides to "duck" down south for a few days.

And then there are days like these.

On days like these all the lights are green and the traffic merges seamlessly. On days like these nothing is too much trouble for anyone, I smile broadly at everyone I meet, and they smile back.

On days like these a new supermarket checkout opens just as I arrive with my overflowing trolley and the kindly lady behind me offers me a spare bag (I never have enough bags).

On days like these my keys are always where I think I've left them and that child who rarely shows any interest in what I teach suddenly develops some curiosity about other languages and cultures.

On days like these I savour every pocket of joy and celebrate each little victory instead of worrying about what lies ahead.

On days like these I am Tigger rather than Eeyore.

On days like these the sun shines brightly but not too fiercely, and the ocean is crystal clear and turquoise blue under multi-textured winter skies. On days like these I catch my breath as I watch the evening light cast its spell across the sand dunes. On days like these I fall asleep to the sound of the waves crashing on the shore and dream of angels dancing in moonbeams.

On days like these I'm not thinking about what it feels like to be told you have anal cancer.

On days like these I give thanks for the gift of life.

SUE TREDGET

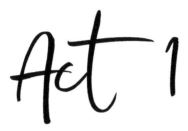

12 March 2021

What's going on?

'You look really good, Sue,' says Pam, my mother-in-law. She hasn't seen me for a while and comments on my weight loss and smart new work clothes.

For some reason I bristle inwardly at the compliment, then feel ungracious for doing so. Pam may be right, I may look good (why do we equate thinness with well-being?) but I haven't been feeling so great lately.

There's no doubt I'd needed to lose weight. When COVID struck, I'd already started losing excess kilos and was determined not to undo my good work during lockdown, to continue fending off the middle-age spread that had slowly but surely begun invading my midriff in recent years. By the beginning of this year, I'd shed about two stone in total – close to 15 kilos – sensibly and gradually, through healthy eating and regular exercise. Eat less, move more, self-discipline, patience. It's not rocket science.

I've stopped off with my in-laws on a weekend trip down south. It's the end of another busy working week, and I'm exhausted. I've been more irritable than usual, impatient, tired a lot of the time, flagging in the afternoons, totally drained by the evening. On too many days, I have to lie down when I get home from school and cannot muster the energy to do anything much for the rest of the day. And there's something niggling at the back of my mind, something I tell myself must be nothing, something I haven't found the strength to do anything about.

I've put my fatigue down to starting a new teaching job in January. A job at a great school where I feel I belong. Fabulous colleagues, excellent department, inspirational headmaster. The perfect place to end my career.

Teaching is tiring at the best of times, but I usually find it invigorating. Now it seems to be wearing me out. I don't understand why I feel so flat. I eat well, exercise daily, rarely drink alcohol. I do all the right things. What's going on?

When I enter the house, my father-in-law, Richard, is lying on his bed, holding a blood-soaked dressing over a wound on his leg. He's been beside himself with frustration for months, following a stroke last November, and has had yet another fall this morning. His mind is still sharp, but his body is in decline. I sit with him on the bed, cross-legged, chat while Pam cleans him up and do what little I can to help before they head off for medical appointments at their retirement village. I continue my journey south filled with sadness and something close to despair. A sense of helplessness and inevitability. Old age. It's brutal.

I do very little over the weekend and sleep a lot. I can't even bring myself to read much. I wanted to do some writing, but nothing flows. I go for walks along the beautiful bay that always stirs my soul but feel a bit blank. The world is tilting strangely. I drive home late on Sunday night and brace myself for another early Monday morning start.

17 March 2021
Upside down

The niggle needs to be dealt with. I take the day off work and make an appointment with Henry, my GP. When I explain why I'm there, he tells me to lie down on the bed. I remove my underwear and turn to the side so he can examine my backside. Henry takes one look at the thing I hoped was nothing and my world turns upside down.

According to the Cancer Council of WA, on any given day 33 West Australians are diagnosed with cancer. Today, on St Patrick's Day of all days, I am one of them.

24 March 2021
Cancer where the sun don't shine

7.15 am
So here I am sitting in the main reception at St John of God Hospital in Subiaco, Western Australia, waiting for my paperwork to be completed, waiting to be admitted for surgery, thinking about all the people I know who have had cancer, those who have survived and those who have not, and wondering which category I'll be in. Thinking about families wracked by grief and loss, of children left motherless or fatherless, of husbands now alone, of wives reinventing themselves after bereavement.

It's been a while since I first felt a small lump when I wiped my backside. I thought it was a haemorrhoid. I had them after giving birth.

I tried to put it out of my mind and tell myself there was no cause for alarm. But it was there every time I went to the toilet, and it wasn't going away. One day I noticed a bit of blood. I tried not to think anything of it for a while longer. I said nothing to Ian, my husband, or to anyone else. Then it got a bit bigger. It was time to pull my head out of the sand.

Over the years, I've occasionally been to see Henry to have lumps checked under my arms and they've always turned out to be cysts. I've usually felt a bit guilty for taking up his time for no reason.

This was not a cyst. This was something far more sinister.

Henry has looked after our family since we moved to Australia in 1999. He has vaccinated, soothed and stitched up my boys, cared for them through infancy, childhood, adolescence and into early manhood. He has listened to my menopausal rantings. He has cheered me up with his no-nonsense approach as I battled depression and anxiety. For over 20 years, Henry has done my PAP smears, checked my weight and blood pressure, sent me for tests, written prescriptions, inspected my sporting injuries. He has referred me to physiotherapists, dermatologists, neurologists. All the usual stuff. Henry is a great family doctor. Henry knows me well. Henry was worried.

He picked up the phone and called a backside surgeon. If Henry was right, this wasn't a form of cancer made commonplace by awareness campaigns. I'd never heard of anyone having cancer in this particular body part. I was flooded with discomfort, fear, anger, disbelief and shock. The indignity of it all. The messiness. Is it shame I feel? Embarrassment? Why should I be ashamed or embarrassed to have cancer of the backside?

When I was at school a friend's mother died from breast cancer, but no one knew what it was until later. Even then, the words were barely whispered, such was the shame, the stigma.

I remember the deep shame that threatened to consume me when I battled depression and anxiety several years ago, the sense of disappearing, of slipping away, of not knowing where I had gone and fearing I would never come back. Of not wanting to be a person who needed to hide away, so great was my guilt at not being able to cope. Of knowing my children deserved a better mother than me and being ashamed of what I had become. Of not wanting to face Ian knowing I must be such a terrible disappointment to him. Of no longer recognising myself.

Eventually I found my way back from darkness to light, but I can never take my mental health for granted. Anxiety still swirls around me, a familiar but unwelcome daily companion. But I survived. And now this? A whole new battle to fight.

'It's hard to get an appointment,' Henry said, as he waited for the phone to be answered. 'But I'll do what I can.'

I heard the muffled sound of someone picking up the phone. Henry spoke clearly and concisely, communicating the urgency of the situation and requesting an appointment as soon as possible. His insistence had the desired effect and I was booked in for the next day.

When I emerged from Henry's room, his receptionist could tell the news wasn't good as I signed the Medicare form.

'I think I have cancer,' I said. 'I can't believe it. It doesn't make any sense.'

'Oh Sue, I'm so sorry,' said Jean, coming to the front of her desk to give me a big hug. She held me tight while I sobbed, offering to drive me home, to call Ian, to do anything she could to help. As I tried to compose myself, she sat beside me and held my hand between both of hers.

'You're a strong woman,' she kept telling me. 'And you have a beautiful family. You'll get through this.'

I hadn't told Ian about either the lump or the appointment. Perhaps because I didn't want to worry him, or because talking about it would make it more real somehow. When I got home I called him at work.

'Please come home now,' I said.

I don't know what's worse. Finding out your spouse has cancer or being the one with the cancer. Still in shock, I was trembling all over as I told him the news.

'I'm so scared,' I kept saying. 'I'm not ready to die yet.'

'Let's not jump the gun until we've seen the specialist,' said Ian, trying to stay calm.

His attempts to reassure me didn't help. I could see the fear in his eyes mirroring my own. And there was no doubt in my mind that Henry had known exactly what he was looking at.

The rest of that day is a complete blur. I have no idea what we did, except that I cried a lot and was more frightened that I'd ever been in my life.

The following day, Ian and I met with a colorectal surgeon called Charles (here in Australia it's normal for patients to call doctors by their first name, no matter where they are on the medical hierarchy) for further investigation. It didn't take long for him to confirm that Henry was right.

'You have cancer of the anal canal.'

I could barely process his words.

Despite the horror of the situation, I liked Charles. His manner was engaging and warm, striking an easy balance between competence and compassion. He was reassuring, but not unrealistically so. He thought the cancer was treatable and booked me in for surgery the following week. What would happen after that would depend on what exactly he found down there. Radiotherapy and chemotherapy were likely.

Back home, my phone kept ringing. Nurses and administrators following up, scheduling scans, checking my personal details again and again. Everyone was kind and friendly but already I was feeling overwhelmed. It was all happening so quickly.

I had the scans yesterday. Three hours in radiology for a PET scan, followed by a CT scan. I was well looked after, wrapped up in warm blankets against the necessary chill of the clinic. I felt as comfortable as I could while also experiencing a slight out of body sensation as I glided into a piece of medical equipment I'd only ever seen on TV.

7.55 am

I've been moved from the main reception to room 14 in Ward 40. It's exactly a week since I saw my GP. The hospital admission process was fast and efficient, the receptionist smiling and warm. My nurse for the morning is called Claudia. She'll be giving me an enema very soon. I have a room of my own. It's comfortable and clean.

8.28 am

The enema has been administered and has done its job, but not completely, I think. I don't feel fully flushed out, so to speak. I'm waiting for further emissions.

Over the last week my mind has been all over the place. It's a real head fuck, this cancer diagnosis thing. One minute I'm telling myself I've got this, I'm strong, I'll pull through. The next I'm cracking jokes about, well, my crack, telling Ian it's no wonder I have anal cancer, I've been married to a real pain in the arse for more than 30 years. I'm making quips about how I've always been a bit different, never followed the crowd, no run-of-the-mill breast cancer for me. And then I'm planning the music for my funeral. I'm thinking of something Irish – Snow Patrol might feature. *Don't You Forget about Me* by Simple Minds at the end, perhaps. Something classical too, soaring strings come to mind. And some stirring, anthemic choral music.

I'm composing letters in my mind to my closest friends across the globe, telling them how much I love them, how much they've enhanced my life with all the joy we've shared. And how they've made life bearable through the bleak times and disappointments. How their spirit is with me now, as I start this journey.

I'm also composing letters in my mind to people who aren't my friends. Does that make me a bad person? I'm mind-drafting words that speak my truth, that don't put other people's feelings and comfort ahead of my reality. I've never been able to do that; Brené Brown tells me I should. Perhaps I should leave these thoughts for another day. But there's something about this diagnosis that makes me want to tell a few things as they are, to stop holding back.

Holding back is what I was taught to do. My mother's lifelong phobia about doctors and hospitals also taught me to be afraid of all things medical. Am I afraid of this? Most certainly. I've been mightily pissed-off too, as well as afraid. And sad. Very, very sad.

I'm not ready to die. There is so much still to do. When I was depressed, I almost lost the will to live. I stared into the abyss and nearly jumped in. Now I have cancer, life seems like the most precious and beautiful thing. I'm sad, but not depressed.

I wonder what kind of cancer patient I'll be. I'm not so sure I'll be one of those gracious, all-loving, all-forgiving sufferers. Will I sail through treatment accepting my fate with dignity and benevolence? Will I be transformed by the trauma into some kind of saint-like being? In my dreams, perhaps. Reality might be a little murkier.

And the irony, oh the irony. I'm fitter than I've been for a long time. I'm proud of my disciplined exercise regime. I walk for at least an hour each day. I'm not overweight. I wanted to be a fit, trim and healthy old lady. Now I'm not so sure I'll get to be any shape of old lady.

I weigh less than I did when I was 18 and I've been feeling much better for it. I don't smoke, very rarely drink these days and never eat junk food. I follow, by and large, a Mediterranean diet. I practise yoga and mindfulness and meditate several times a week. I swim in the ocean and walk on the beach and marvel at sunsets and the glory of nature.

So, go figure. What's this all about, this goddamn cancerous thing that has invaded my body? Why me? Not fair. Not fair. *Not fair*. Why do good people have to suffer, and bad people get away with murder?

My nurse this morning is so lovely. She keeps saying sorry. Sorry I have to do this enema. Sorry you can't have a cup of tea. She's a delight. Nurses are amazing.

More positives. I'm in Perth, Western Australia, probably the best place in the world to be during this accursed pandemic if you need urgent medical care. To the best of my knowledge, there are no COVID patients in this hospital. There is no more pressure than usual on doctors and nurses. My referral was swift, appointments made without delay. This means, I realise, that my situation is urgent. But my friends in the UK tell me cancer patients there are not so fortunate, if fortunate is the word.

9.55 am

A different nurse appears. It's time to go to the holding bay. I undress and don my hospital gown, sexy cap and some very tight stockings to prevent blood clots. I'm wheeled through the hospital on my bed and parked beside someone called

Antoinette who tells her nurse she doesn't like to be called Toni.

'What about Toni Collette,' I say to the complete stranger lying next to me. She and her nurse laugh. *You're terrible Muriel*, I want to add, but hold back.

I close my eyes against the bright, bright light. It feels very cold. Another nurse goes through my details, yet again, to make sure I am who I should be. I close my eyes again for a while. My lovely backside surgeon comes for a reassuring chat, accompanied by another doctor called Kevin. As the procedure is explained, to make sure I understand, Kevin nods empathetically, or at least I think he does. I can't see his facial features very well without my glasses. I bombard Charles with questions. I have so many questions.

'One thing at a time,' he says.

Jennifer, my anaesthetist, arrives. Suddenly I'm freezing cold and my whole body starts to tremble. A nurse wraps me in a warm blanket. I feel cocooned and cared for.

Jennifer searches in vain for a vein (boom boom) in my left arm and it hurts. My right arm is bruised and battered from yesterday's needles and that tube thing they put in to administer the pre-scan stuff.

'I bruise very easily,' I tell her.

'I can see that. Your veins are very small,' she says, before she finally succeeds.

'Is it in now?' I ask, resisting the urge to add 'said the actress to the bishop'. Ben, my youngest, picked up this phrase when I said it at home recently and found it hilarious. I don't think people say it anymore. When Ben tried it out with his friends, they had no idea what he was talking about. Apparently there's a modern equivalent, which now evades me and is much less amusing.

'Yes,' she says. 'It's in. I'll give you something to help you relax.'

I go to some lovely place and time stands still.

24 March 2021
Tea and sandwiches

11.55 am

I open my eyes and I'm back in Room 14. I feel strange and floaty and rather nice. A nurse comes in and I talk gibberish to her. I like this feeling. It's peaceful. I savour the floating sensation for a while longer.

Somehow, I find my phone and call both Ian and Ben and talk gibberish to them, too.

Another staff member comes to see if I'd like some sandwiches and a cup of tea. I realise I'm ravenous. I ask for strong white tea and it arrives with a plate of perfectly cut, de-crusted sandwiches. The tea is hot and delicious. The sandwiches taste divine. I compliment the refreshment provider on her amazing tea making, just as I like it.

I call my sister-in-law, Anne, who has flown over from Sydney to visit her dad. She had breast cancer a couple of years ago, as did her older sister, Jane, at the end of last year, and their mother, 27 years ago. So much cancer. It's crazy. But they all survived. I hope I do too.

I'm still talking gibberish and Anne laughs. I tell her to look after Ian and my boys if I don't make it. 'Oh Suze,' she says, and I cry. She's awesome.

1.25 pm

It's lunch time and when I'm offered more food I opt for more perfectly cut sandwiches and tea rather than roast beef. I devour them. Who knew hospital food was so yummy?

I call my friend Marita who lives in Melbourne and works for BCNA – the Breast Cancer Network of Australia. She can't believe my news. And she's never heard of anal cancer. Everyone knows about breast cancer, but cancer of the anal canal is most definitely not in the public consciousness.

'Fuck,' she says.

'Yes, fuck,' I say.

It's such a comfort to hear her voice. Marita knows what it's like, the whole cancer journey thing. She won't dress it up or shirk the awfulness of it. She'll be right there, with me all the way. We plan to meet when this is all over. It's been too long. COVID has made it too long. As soon as we can fly across the country again without risking lockdowns, we'll make it happen. I need things to look forward to.

2.35 pm

Kevin arrives. He's Irish, I realise. From County Mayo, I discover. I seem to be very chatty in hospital.

'Do you know Achill Island?' I ask. Achill is a wild and beautiful island off the coast of Mayo.

'I know it well,' he replies.

I tell him that Achill is where my Mum and Dad met, and it's where I learnt to swim. Not many people know about it.

Kevin tells me the surgery was a success, there were no surprises, and I can go home today, rather than stay overnight as originally booked. They didn't need to excise the tumour, which is apparently a good thing. I thought it would be better to get it out. I think the plan now is to blast the hell out of it with chemotherapy and radiotherapy.

'Is the lovely backside surgeon not coming back to see me?' I ask.

Kevin tells me I'll see him next week when we discuss the treatment. He can't discuss the details of that until the oncology team has met on Monday. We chat a little more and he wishes me all the best.

I think I doze for a while and then Charles does indeed appear. I'm so pleased to see him. I trust this man implicitly. How can that be? He reiterates what Kevin said, that all went smoothly, the tumour is malignant but didn't need to be removed. He has the PET and CT scan results and the news is encouraging. The cancer doesn't seem to have spread anywhere else. The tumour seems localised and can be treated with chemotherapy and radiotherapy. The success rate is good.

I want to reach out and hold his hand, but refrain. Instead, I thank him profusely for coming to see me. He explains that he knew I was anxious (anxious, moi?) and wanted to tell me personally. He'll see me next week in his rooms to discuss the treatment. He doesn't have the precise details yet but tells me it will be tailored specifically for me and my type of cancer.

I message Ian and he replies with a line full of heart emojis and the one with the party streamers.

A nurse called Sharon arrives, my special cancer nurse. She called me at home a few days ago for a chat and said she'd see me in hospital. She sits down and goes through the treatment plan. She has a gracious, calm manner but pulls no punches. I like people who are real. Sharon is real.

My treatment will start with a week of chemotherapy, radiotherapy every day for six weeks, and then another week of chemotherapy, which, apparently, I'll do at home. I'll have it administered through a pump attached to PICC line – a peripherally inserted central catheter – which will be put in place before treatment starts.

'So you're telling me I'll be walking around with a pump full of chemotherapy drugs everywhere I go?' I ask her, somewhat alarmed.

'Yes, exactly. It means you don't have to sit in hospital for hours to have your chemotherapy,' she explains.

'How big is this pump? What does it look like?' I ask her, unable to visualise such a contraption.

'It's not that big. You can put it in your pocket or your handbag,' she answers.

I'm astonished.

We move on and talk about work. Sharon advises taking time off for the duration of the treatment.

'It can be gruelling and you're likely to be very tired,' she says, before going through all the potential side-effects, which I really don't want to hear about.

'I don't care,' I say, 'as long as it works.'

I think about work. I'll have to take leave without pay as I don't have any sick leave. I spoke to my HR manager last week to tell him my news, and before I said too much, he stopped me in my tracks.

'Sue, you don't have to give me any details. Your job is safe. It's our role to support you through this and we will. Whether you've been here 10 minutes or 10 years, we will treat you just the same. We are very glad to have you here. You are a highly valued member of staff. Take as much leave as you need. We'll work it out. Leave that to us. Your health is the most important thing.'

I know he was simply telling me what all good employers should, but I also know that not all employers do what they should. He's from Belfast, my HR manager. Unlike me, he hasn't lost any of his accent. Only someone with Henry Higgins-esque linguistic skills could detect mine now, although it's still alive and well, among the mishmash of English and Australian sounds. He's been in Australia for over 20 years but sounds as though he's never strayed very far from the Falls Road. He sounds like home.

Now, I remember his words as I listen to Sharon and resolve to break the habit of a lifetime and stop worrying about work or pay or mortgages or superannuation. Well, I'm going to try. I need to focus on my health and give myself the best chance of recovery. Having daily radiotherapy on top of a full workload and walking around school with a pump full of chemotherapy drugs don't seem like feasible options. I'm not going to get any awards for so-called bravery.

Years ago, I taught in a school where a senior staff member worked throughout her cancer treatment. She was held up as an example of resilience and fortitude, lauded in front of the whole school as a superhuman for her dedication, commitment and unfaltering service. It made the rest of us feel bad for taking a day or two off if we had a cold or a migraine, or any other kind of regular ailment for which we were perfectly entitled to take time off.

Taking sick leave has long had a weird stigma in the workplace, I've found. It's a lot better now that COVID has made it our duty to stay at home if we are unwell. It has become much less frowned upon. It only took a global pandemic for that to happen.

Teaching is tiring at the best of times. Standing in front of a class of 15-year-olds, managing their learning, their behaviour and their differing needs requires an enormous amount of energy. Energy I need to conserve.

Sharon gives me her card, which includes her mobile number, and says I can contact her anytime.

I call Ian to come and pick me up. The afternoon nurse signs me off for departure. I get dressed, check I have everything, leave the room, walk down the stairs with my now redundant overnight case to the second floor of the hospital and out through the main reception. I walk for about 10 minutes, wheeling my case behind me, to a fruit and vegetable shop where I've arranged to meet Ian. I had surgery under general anaesthetic a few hours ago, I have cancer, but I feel pretty good. I fill my basket with mangoes, pomegranates, bananas and all manner of leafy goodness.

I get to the checkout and realise I have no idea where my overnight case is. The case with my MacBook in it. Ian suddenly appears beside me as I calmly tell the cashier I can't find my case and ask if anyone has seen it. Ian searches the store before spotting it by the entrance, beside all the shopping trolleys.

'I guess the anaesthetic hasn't completely worn off,' I say to him, strangely unperturbed.

We drive home.

'I was planning the music for my funeral this morning,' I tell Ian.

'And I was composing my speech for your funeral,' he replies. What are we like?

Once home, I put down my stuff, unpack the food, greet the dog, and start to chop vegetables for a stir-fry while I call Anne to give her an update. She's relieved to hear all went as well as it could today. She knows it won't be easy.

I call a work colleague to fill her in on my day and we chat for ages about not very much. We both studied languages and did our teaching diplomas at the same universities in the UK. Small world.

Marita messages again. She's still in shock.

'Hi Suze, how the fuck did this happen?' she writes. She's fond of swearing, my friend Marita, as am I when needs must. There are times when nothing less than an expletive will do. (I was heartened to read recently that the judicious use of swear words is a sign of intelligence.)

'Why do terrible things happen to the best of people?' she wonders, again.

She tells me she's been googling and can find hardly anything about anal cancer. Except that it's quite rare and affects more women than men.

'You know me,' I message back. 'I've never liked to follow the crowd.'

She sends me the laughing emoji and we message back and forward for a while, finishing with 'love you' and 'ditto'. She lights up my life.

I look outside and watch the setting sun, our windows creating the perfect picture frame for the deep orange glow that fills the sky. The sun slips quietly below the horizon. It will rise again tomorrow, and life will go on.

25 March 2021
Climb every mountain

8.30 am
How strange. I slept well without any medication. I'm not in pain, just a little uncomfortable in the nether regions. I wonder how many euphemisms I can use for the part of my body that

has morphed. Every time I speak or write the word 'anal' I feel uncomfortable. It's not a pleasant word, anal. Maybe I just need to keep saying it to normalise it, rather than treating it as the body part that shall not be named.

After the sun set last night, my mother-in-law called, relieved to hear that my scans were encouraging. I tell her I'm not out of the woods yet. There's a long road ahead. I don't want to be falsely hopeful, unrealistically positive. She tells me she knows I'll be OK. *How does she know that?* I think. No-one can know I'm going to be OK. I feel bad that I can't mirror her relief. I don't really feel relief. I just feel less despair. She's been through a lot lately with both her daughters' breast cancer and her husband's declining health and need for constant care. She bears it all stoically but she's exhausted. She needs me to get better. I try my best to sound more upbeat than I feel.

10.19 am

I don't know what to do with myself. I can't do much exercise, apparently. I can go for gentle walks, but one of the nurses in the ward told me not to do my daily weights and stretches when I asked her advice. Exercise is one of my essentials for sanity. So is swimming in the ocean. She told me not to do that either. I'm not sure why. Isn't saltwater a natural cleanser?

I feel anxious and worried about work, despite my resolution yesterday. I'm coming and going in and out of so many different emotions, from one moment to the next. I check some work emails about reports and deadlines and parent-teacher interviews next week. I don't know if I can face those. Private school parents can be tough. I don't want to break down in the middle of a discussion about Johnny's lack of application or Joseph's gaming tendencies.

I watch the French news for 10 minutes and then switch off. Europe is in turmoil. I keep telling myself that Western Australia is the best place in the world to have cancer in the time of COVID.

My surgeon's receptionist calls. They are expecting the biopsy results on Monday. We book an appointment for next Tuesday. She asks how I am. I tell her I'm a bit anxious (understatement of the year).

'That's understandable,' she says.

I'm playing a waiting game again and I'm not very good at it. I don't know the rules. Are there any rules? Do I make up my own? Do I override the medical certificate I was given and go back to work tomorrow? I'm pacing around the house, unable to settle to anything much.

11.55 am

A senior colleague returns my call from earlier this morning. I want to keep them updated and be transparent about all of this. When I give him the cold, hard facts he's beyond understanding. I must do whatever I need to do, and the school will support me. My health must come first. People keep telling me this. Have I not put my health first often enough? I wonder. Have I done things even when I felt tired, drained, stressed, anxious, when my body needed a break, when my mind needed to refresh? Haven't we all? Don't we all?

Earlier, I chatted to one of the HR staff about leave and pay and processes and who to tell and how. She impressed on me, again, that the school would be there to support me.

'We're a beautiful community,' she said.

I've certainly felt that. I like this new school and I must have faith. People seem to walk their talk. Words don't seem empty.

People greet you. Everyone is friendly. Teaching is tough and, sadly, the working environment can make it even tougher if there isn't sufficient support, kindness, decency, humanity. I've experienced the lack thereof myself and heard many stories of bullying and burnout. I'm at the tail-end of my career and I want to end it well. I want to keep teaching here in this caring, close-knit community for a little while longer.

The surgeon calls to say he has received the results and the malignancy is confirmed. We all knew, but now we have the clinical evidence. He will see me next week, and in the meantime I should expect calls from two different oncologists – one for radiotherapy and one for chemotherapy – to talk about the treatment. And from someone else to arrange a colonoscopy as an additional precaution, given the location of my tumour.

It's all a bit confusing. Everything is moving so fast. So many doctors are involved. I'm already forgetting who does what. I suddenly feel completely overwhelmed and start to cry, sucking in deep gulps of air in an attempt to stem the tears. I give up and let them flow until I'm all cried out.

Later, the colonoscopy receptionist calls to book me in, for three weeks hence.

'It seems too long to wait,' I tell her.

She puts me on hold and comes back with an appointment for Monday, in a few days' time. I think that might be too soon, given that I've just had surgery.

'I'm seeing the surgeon again on Tuesday,' I tell her. 'Does he need to examine me first, before the colonoscopy?'

She's not sure – she'll check with him tomorrow and call me back. More waiting and wondering. My energy plummets.

The Alliance Française Film Festival is in town, and I suddenly decide to take myself off to the cinema in the middle of the day to stop myself going crazy, and just because I can. The film's not great, but it's French and it takes me out of my head for a while. A middle-aged woman finds out her middle-aged husband is having an affair with their son's not middle-aged teacher. *Très français.*

I nearly fall asleep at one point but it passes two hours. The cinema is close to school, so I'll go there afterwards to collect some assessments to mark. I'm foolish, perhaps, picking up marking when I should be resting. But I'll be going to school tomorrow and I want to have the test marks ready and entered into the system and be able to give my students meaningful feedback. I want to end the week feeling I've achieved something other than getting through the start of this cancer journey. I'm trying to think of it as an adventure, but today it's a soaring peak whose summit I'll never reach, the hardest trek of my life. I'm not even at base camp. Not even close.

I need to phone a friend. I call Lorna in the UK. We don't speak often, but always pick up as if we'd seen each other yesterday. She's calm when I tell her my news, upset for me, but calm, which is what I need. She doesn't bombard me with questions, instinctively knowing that would be the last thing I need in my still shocked and very delicate state. I feel warm and cosy inside when I talk to Lorna. We love each other and always tell each other so. She'll be right there, with me all the way, even from afar. I have the best friends. Quality, not quantity. I'll savour each conversation and harness the love. I'll channel their faith in me, their care for me. I'll carry the precious gift of friendship to the summit of this mountain.

10.15 pm

I'm tired now. I should be in bed, but my mind is racing. I've marked the test, entered the data, filled in the feedback, uploaded the documents. There's so much to do in teaching these days. We're always feeding back and uploading and reflecting. It can be exhausting. I'll go to work tomorrow, and then it's the weekend. After that, who knows?

People might look at me differently, now they know I have cancer. I don't think I look any different. This is what cancer looks like. A fairly fit if somewhat haggard, slightly frazzled middle-aged woman. I have cancer, but I am not cancer. I am still me.

Bed beckons. I'll warm my heat pack and curl myself around it. Tomorrow is another day. One step at a time.

26 March 2021

When you wish upon a star

Some ungodly hour

When I had depression all I had to do was take a small white pill every day for a year and lie around on the sofa watching Rick Stein food shows on repeat, taking nothing in. There wasn't anything wrong with my body, but it felt as though I'd lost my mind, like I'd never feel anything except despair ever again. I didn't want to be here. I didn't want to be alive.

Now I have cancer, I'll have tubes and needles and pain and daily trips to hospital and nausea and fatigue. I've been shown the pages and pages of potential risks and side-effects. Now I have cancer I fiercely, madly, deeply want to stay alive. I'd walk through fire to stay alive. I'll take the tubes up my backside, I'll put up with whatever needs to be done if I can stay alive.

Am I a bad person? Is that why I have cancer?

How come I have cancer and can still feel joy?

How come I can hold a plank for five minutes and walk for hours and still have cancer?

Late last night I chatted to our elder son Daniel, who's been living in London since 2017. Ian told him about my diagnosis yesterday. We're so far away and international travel is not an option at present. We'd have to fill in forms and jump through numerous hoops to get him here. And even if travel were approved, he'd have to quarantine in a hotel for two weeks at his own expense. I understand the need to quarantine, but why can't people do it at home? Why are people financially penalised for wanting to be with family, particularly family who are sick? But then again, thanks to the state government's policies, I can have cancer treatment without delay in a COVID-free hospital. The Premier's sword is double-edged.

I'm missing Daniel so much. My Danny Boy. I used to sing that Irish anthem to him as a baby. I used to play him all kinds of music when he was growing up. I remember sometimes playing the Oasis album, *What's the Story Morning Glory*, probably at far too high a volume, when he was crying, which wasn't often. He was a very happy baby. Within no time, Liam's less than dulcet tones would lull him into slumber.

Now Daniel is a musician in London. He still loves Oasis and the estranged Gallagher brothers. He thinks Liam lives in his neighbourhood, after passing the parka-clad self-appointed rock god in the street one day.

'You should have spoken to him,' I said.

'I'm sure he'd have told me to fuck off,' Daniel replied. He's probably right.

We haven't seen Daniel for over a year. He has a new track, *Stray Star*, out today on Spotify. It makes me cry every time I listen to it. He's always been a stray star, dancing to the beat of a different drum.

Daniel writes catchy melodies and lyrics that are heart-wrenching one minute and uplifting the next, but it's tough to make it as a musician in this 15-second-attention-span world. Everything is so fast and furious. It's more about your Insta grid than any musical talent. Social media isn't Daniel's thing. Self-promotion doesn't come naturally to him. He doesn't have a single narcissistic bone in his body. He's an artist, a poet. He needs a lucky break.

When Daniel was a baby, we used to hold him by the window so he could look up at the stars before bedtime. He'd put his little feet in his little socks on the windowsill and we'd point out the brightest star in the sky and call it his Lucky Star. Every night he'd look up at the sky and find his Lucky Star. If it was cloudy (which was often in the north-east of England, where we lived then) we'd try to imagine which cloud it was hiding behind. Right now, I'm thinking of Daniel, my stray star. I'm holding him tight in my heart and wishing on that Lucky Star for all of us. For me to heal. For someone with influence to notice his music amid the white noise. For the world to return to a place where we can be together again, at least once each year.

Daniel's music will help to carry me through this.

Ben still lives at home with us. I can hug him every day and gain strength from his belief that I will be well again. Both my boys are great huggers.

Time stretches ahead. Uncertainty swirls. Maybe I'll become addicted to online shopping. The only things I've ever ordered online are books and one pair of trainers in a style I already had. It scares me, the filling of a virtual shopping cart. I can see it would easily get out of control. And I've heard that online shoppers in search of a bargain are easy fodder for scammers.

How did I get to be here, writing in the middle of the night?

It's the only thing I know how to do. Well, not the only thing, but it makes me feel good, even when writing about confronting things. It makes them seem more normal, part of the messiness of life. It chips away at the awfulness of it all, releases some of the fear, helps me to accept the reality. Words helped me write my way out of depression. Now I'm writing my way through cancer. Ironically, this heinous invasion of my body is giving me more time to do the thing I love.

I'm not yet sure what I'll do with this writing. It seems too long to post as blogs on my website, or on my Facebook page: *Hey guys, I have cancer and yes, I'd love your feedback.*

Before March 17, I was 45,000 words into my first novel. On the days when it flows it feels amazing, but it's been a stop-start process from the get-go. No Stephen King-like disciplined writing routine for me. I'll suddenly be inspired one weekend and write for hours, and then do nothing for weeks. I think it scares me a bit. That's a common writer's thing, fear. Just ask Elizabeth Gilbert, or Marian Keyes.

I'm not sure fiction is my genre. I find myself writing about people I know and giving them different names, changing their jobs and where they live. Maybe all writers do that to some extent.

7.08 am
Sleep eluded me. Coffee's been drunk. I'm going to get ready for work. Breathe Sue, breathe.

26 March 2021
One day at a time

4.58 pm
Every Friday, at my school, we have an hour-long assembly. My school does assembly like no other I've worked in. There's a genuine appreciation of ritual, tradition and heritage that resonates deeply in my soul. To commence proceedings, students march to the beat of a pipe band dressed in full highland regalia. It's

more Scottish than Scotland. I love it. There's beautiful music and stirring hymn singing and solemn praying and thought-provoking speeches. Awards are given and received, achievement celebrated, but always with humility. Effort and decency are valued just as much as winning. I really notice that at this school. Victories aren't trumpeted. They are acknowledged with grace and boy does the world needs more grace. It's nice to find it here.

I make it to school this morning and line up to process into the hall with the other staff. The headmaster spots me and walks my way. He left a message on my phone yesterday, telling me he'd heard my news.

'Let me know if there's anything we can do,' he said.

Today he checks that I received his message. I had called back but was put through to his PA's voicemail. He's a busy man. Now, we have a short but heartfelt exchange and I get the strong sense that he has my back. I felt it three years ago when I worked here as a relief teacher. This school is special. It has a tangible sense of community. Much of this, I feel, is due to the headmaster, the tone he sets and the staff he appoints.

Today, one of the student leaders gives an update on the Greatest Shave fundraiser, an annual event here in WA. The students have raised in the region of $50,000 for leukaemia research, maybe more. Another student walks onto the stage and an interview is set up. The boy is a leukaemia survivor. He speaks clearly and frankly about his diagnosis at the age of nine, the months of treatment, his feelings, the support from family and friends, his amazing medical team. He's now three years clear of cancer.

I'm deeply moved. I'm not alone, I think. I'm one of millions dealing with cancer in this country. And how wonderful that we're listening to this in a school assembly, and you could hear a pin drop.

The assembly ends, as always, with a rousing rendition of the school song, which I find oddly comforting. I head to my classroom. It's lovely to see my Year 11s. They're full of life and character and fun and chat. I tell them I was pleased with their assessment results and we go through the marks and discuss the feedback. It's nice. I like teaching these students. They look like young adults but they're still just kids really. I laugh at their jokes, their funny sayings, their adolescent humour and love of banter. They must think I'm ancient. *Retain your childlike enthusiasm*, I want to say to them. *Never lose touch with your inner child. Don't grow up too quickly.*

After the lesson I sit quietly in my classroom for a while. The hospital calls to confirm the colonoscopy for Monday. They've checked with the surgeon and he wants it done then. So that's good, I guess. Less waiting. Get it over and done with. The receptionist talks me through the three days of preparation. Not much dietary pleasure for me over the weekend.

7.45 pm
I go for a gentle walk. The evening air is fragrant and restoring as I stroll through the fading light.

I notice the smell of the frangipanis outside my front door, the melodic chords in a favourite song through my headphones, the chirping of the crickets, the evening birdsong. I notice everything and I feel joy. How can that be? I'm clinging to these moments of joy.

I've just realised that all the women in my husband's life have had cancer. His mother, my mother, his two sisters and me. What's that all about? Can the guy not get a break?

This is life and life is messy. Sickness and sadness are part of being human. I have to believe I'll get through this. One day at a time.

27 March 2021

I'll get by with a little help from my friends

9.30 pm

Today disappeared in a searing migraine that struck in the early hours and only lifted when the sky was streaked with the pink and orange of an autumn sunset. Head splitting pain, nausea, vomiting, the lot. As if I won't have enough of this when I start chemotherapy. Was it a warning of what's to come, my mind anticipating the trials ahead? Ian tells me it was a normal bodily response after a week of immense strain coming to terms with my new reality.

I'm prepping for the colonoscopy on Monday, so am only allowed a restricted diet today. I guess being wiped out for more than 12 hours made that easy. Tomorrow it's total fasting, clear fluids only. I ate some white bread and boiled eggs this evening, two of the options on the diet sheet, and won't eat again until Monday night.

I had a long chat with Jess, another friend in the UK, when I resurfaced today. I'd sent her what I've written so far and asked for her feedback. I'm wondering about starting a cancer blog but it seems so raw. I'm not sure I'm ready to share my vulnerability with the world.

Is it too much, too honest, too confronting? Who would want to read about my experience with cancer?

'That doesn't matter,' said Marita, another recipient of the story thus far. 'Who cares what other people think? Your friends will read it. I want to know how you are, I want to follow your progress. I'm here with you all the way, and you must do things your way. People can read it if they want, or not, or check in now and again and you can still have one-on-one chats with friends, the friends who lift you up.'

I'm still not sure I want to document all this publicly. It seems to be taking on a life of its own. Somewhere in the back of my mind it's starting to feel more like a book than a blog.

Marita is a big supporter of my writing; I finished my first book sitting in her apartment in Melbourne. When it was published, she shared it with her book club and arranged for me to be there when they discussed it, talk to them about the process of writing it and answer their questions. I felt like a real author, flying across the country to meet my readers.

Jess told me she's worried about my need to always be doing something. She thinks it isn't good for me to be so busy, that at this stage in our lives we need to reflect and step back and slow down. She wondered if I should still be working so much. It came across very clearly in the writing, she said, my drive to be achieving, to always be accomplishing something.

Jess is one of my closest friends, but I felt a bit attacked. And therefore defensive. This was not what I needed to hear. I enjoy working. I still love teaching. I like to achieve things. Having a purpose in life is very important for good mental health. I'm still reeling from my diagnosis and don't have the energy to counter what she says and respond as I would wish. I feel rattled, unsettled. It didn't help that she also questioned the need for chemotherapy. She's not a fan of western medicine and rarely goes to the doctor.

As Jess talked, I wished I hadn't shared what I'd written. She mentioned that I still appear wounded by past events and urged me to be gentle with myself. I know she cares about me and always means well, even if our views on modern medicine don't align, and she's right about my old wounds. I'm aware that revisiting the past isn't always helpful, but sometimes scars resurface.

We talked about her study of Buddhism and the lessons it teaches, and reflected on work and people and family and friends. She kept telling me that I must be kind to myself.

'I'm trying,' I said. 'I'm trying.'

Jess challenges me and we don't always agree. She ended the call by telling me how happy she was to have had me as her friend all these years. The feeling is mutual. But I'm concerned that I can't confide in her as I would like, and confused that I should feel this way about one of my closest friends.

I exchange messages with more friends and feel their love, from near and far.

A while later, I call Georgia, another friend in the UK. She's rocked by my news but has absolute faith in me. These phone calls are so precious. They've sustained me through COVID and will continue to sustain me through this new challenge.

Georgia has good news about the flat she's been trying to buy for months. It's been a protracted process, with hurdles appearing each time she thought the deal was done, but she loved the flat and persisted. It's about 10 minutes' walk from Daniel's place in north London. I'm planning to visit as soon as COVID (and cancer) allows. The flat has two bedrooms and she calls one of them mine. I tell her just how want my bedroom to be, and we laugh. I need things to look forward to. I'll get by with a little help from my friends.

Georgia is a journalist and novelist, and we discuss writing and possibilities. She understands the power of words, the creative drive. I tell her about my lovely website guy, Fred, who sent me the most beautiful message yesterday when I emailed to tell him my news and ask for advice. He's going to rework the website with a new section for a blog about all of this. Top bloke, Fred.

Some other nice things happened at school yesterday. The senior colleague I talked to the other day checked in with me before I left – he oversees all the staff absences. I told him I didn't know how I would react to treatment. I may tolerate it well, or not. I may need to take a big chunk of time off, or I may be able to keep teaching.

'We'll play it by ear,' he reassured me. 'That's absolutely fine.'

When I mentioned co-curricular duties, which all staff must do, and the parent-teacher interviews next week, he batted away my concerns.

'Don't even think about it,' he said. 'You're not doing any of that. We'll sort it out.'

He thanked me for being so open and keeping the school informed. Top bloke. A man of genuine compassion and integrity. A reflective man. Men get a lot of bad press these days, but there are plenty of good ones out there.

There were flowers on my desk when I got back to the office. From the languages department, with love.

'We're here for you,' they wrote.

My head of department had marked all my Year 10 tests and entered the data. He's worried for me. I can sense it. He's a man of deep faith and has been praying for me. Another top bloke.

I chatted with a colleague who joined the staff this year with me. After expressing his care and support, he told me the joyous news of his partner's pregnancy.

'How wonderful,' I say. 'I'm so happy for you'.

I love that he shared this with me. I love that he could show his concern, then just treat me normally.

'A quarantine baby,' he then added, with a cheeky grin. 'Not much else to do in lockdown.'

They moved here from Brisbane at the start of the year. Yet another top bloke. Funny, perceptive and kind. I'm thrilled about his impending parenthood. Life goes on. New life will arrive.

It's past midnight now. I slept on and off all day, through the migraine, so I'm up late. The house is quiet. Ben has just come in from a day and night out with friends. Ian and the dog are fast asleep. I'm wondering how I'll get through tomorrow, with only clear fluids to sustain me. I will get through. I have no choice.

29 March 2021
Born to be a stray star

9.00 am
I'm hollowed out and I've only just started the three litres of bowel preparation I need to drink today. Yesterday, it was liquids all day, and the first batch of preparation. Anyone who's had a colonoscopy will know all about this. It's a common procedure. Millions have them on a regular basis. This is my first.

I look in the mirror, briefly. I'm disappearing. My hair needs attention. I was due to have a haircut on Saturday. Personal grooming will have to wait. The possibility of being bald if my hair falls out is confronting. Like Samson, I gain strength from my hair. Looking at a bald woman may be uncomfortable for others, but I'm not going to bother with wigs. I'll wrap colourful scarves around my head or wear funky hats.

I remember that nurse Sharon told me my hair may not necessarily fall out, but I want to get it cut so there is less to fall out if it does happen.

'You'll lose your pubic hair, though,' she said.

Great. No waxing required. I'll be bang on trend, feeling as sexy as a cabbage.

Yesterday
I awake to a YouTube clip Jess has sent me from the London Buddhist centre. I play it through my speaker and stay lying in

bed, coming in and out of consciousness, hearing about particles of light and radiant sun. It's soothing. Ian is out cycling, and Ben is working at his café. The house is Sunday morning quiet. I leave the sliding doors open and hear the distant hum of lawn trimming, of birds singing, dogs barking. Of suburban normality.

I work all morning, preparing things for my Year 12s. It feels satisfying. I need to pass the time and take my mind off the hunger pangs. I want to feel useful and make sure my students stay on track in my absence. I'm wondering about telling them why I've been away. I ran this past the senior colleague I talked to last week.

'Is there a school policy on such things?' I ask him. 'I don't want to burden the boys.'

'Our school states that we prepare students for life, and this is part of life,' he said. 'You must do whatever feels comfortable, and we will support you.'

That word again, support.

I'm hoping to make it to school tomorrow morning, depending on how I feel after the colonoscopy, so I could tell them then. Can I do it, without breaking down? Am I strong enough?

Easter holidays start this week. We were planning a short camping trip and then a stay down south. I was so looking forward to it.

In the afternoon, Anne, Ian's sister, drives up the freeway from her parents' retirement village for a change of scene. She flew over from Sydney a few days ago to try to sort out a care and respite plan for her dad. He's up and down, but mostly down. I'm not much company today, but it's lovely to see her.

Anne and Ian head to the beach. They have a natural, easy brother-sister relationship. Full of love and banter and laughter. I envy it.

Ben joins them at a beach restaurant for dinner, after his first hockey match of the season. I would have been there normally, but I just don't have the strength to see people today. I think about telling the hockey club my news. I might get Ian to do that. I want to keep going to matches, to hang out with the hockey parent crew when I can, but don't want to be fielding too many questions.

I while away the afternoon watching feel-good romantic movies on Amazon Prime while drinking my first batch of colonoscopy preparation. It's disgusting. I enjoy the movies, though. I love a good rom com.

The dinner party returns and Anne heads back to her parents' place. Ian and Ben and I chat a little. I do some posting about Daniel's latest release. I'm his biggest fan. The video for "Stray Star" is out on YouTube, filmed on a shoestring in Muswell Hill, London N10, where I lived in the 1980s and where he lives now, in the very same street where I bought my first property. It's amazing that in a metropolis of more than 10 million people Daniel ends up living a stone's throw from where I lived. He can see my old flat from his window.

I love the video. It makes me smile and cry at the same time. *Born to be a stray star*, he sings. We watch it on the big screen, the sound cranked up. Now we need the world to discover it and make my boy's dreams come true. We're kindred spirits, Daniel and me. The mother-son bond is a beautiful thing. He's got his shit together a lot earlier than I did. He has more equanimity at the tender age of 24 than I have in my 58-year-old big toe.

The day begins to fade. I love the evening light, the softness, the gentle receding into silence. Ian and Ben head to bed. They are early risers most days, for cycling and coffee making. I savour the stillness and prepare for the night. I'll be in and out of sleep, no doubt. I line up some podcasts on my phone, BBC Radio 4, *In Our Time Philosophy*, *The Forum*. Some thought-provoking, intelligent conversation to see me through the night. Tomorrow is another day.

29 March 2021
More tea and sandwiches

10.09 am
I'm drinking my way through the three litres. It doesn't taste too bad. I'm following the instructions to the letter. Two glasses every 20 minutes.

I send a couple of emails, do a little more schoolwork, have a quick look at the French news.

Fred has emailed. He's started the website revamp. I write back with my thoughts.

I see a comment on Instagram from my nephew's medical practice in the UK about Daniel's music. One of his staff is a fan and plays it in the clinic for the patients. My nephew really appreciates her support for Daniel, she writes. My heart swells. Little things, small kindnesses.

I haven't told my brother and sister my news. I don't know how, when or even if I should do that. We process emotion and hurt and pain and grief and all the hard stuff very differently. So much so that for years I was convinced I was adopted (until my husband pointed out that I have mannerisms just like my Mum and do something with my jaw that makes me look just like my brother).

We're not in regular contact, we don't check in daily and keep each other updated on the details of our lives. I'd like it to be different. My brother and sister seem to have become closer since my eldest sister and parents died, which is great but makes me feel a bit excluded. I'm super sensitive about family matters and all too aware of the dangers of familial rabbit holes. It would most definitely not be in my best interests to venture down one now.

I'm not ready to tell them but I will in due course. They have their own busy lives and have had their own challenges to face through COVID and lockdowns. I think I'll know when the time is right. There are lots of people I haven't told. This is pretty confronting news; I don't always want to talk about it and you never quite know how people might react. Writing I can do until the cows come home (especially if I'm not sure anyone will ever read it); talking is another thing entirely. But my siblings are in my thoughts as I navigate my way through this.

3.25 pm

Here we go again. I'm sitting in the admissions area of the hospital for the second time in a week, waiting to go up to the colonoscopy ward. The prospect of another anaesthetic followed by tea and sandwiches awaits. Yay! More floaty feelings.

I managed to drink all the stuff, the litres of preparation liquid, but I'm not fully abluted, yet again. I'm sitting close to the bathroom looking at all the other people who are waiting and wondering what their stories are. Are they, like me, at the start of a mountain climb or just having a routine check?

This morning I posted my cancer news in a Facebook group I belong to. I'm not really into Facebook groups or online (over) sharing, but this one seems like a genuine community, a safe place (I hope), an offshoot of the popular Chat 10 Looks 3 podcast. I'm uplifted by the messages of support and hope, and the survival tales. So many cancer survival tales. It's heartening.

I'm getting used to sitting in waiting rooms. I put on my headphones and try to zone out with a calming playlist. I couldn't live without music. It's one of my key coping mechanisms. Music and nature and writing and exercise will help me through this. Help to process and reflect and articulate. Help me to own it and be comfortable naming it, this new reality of mine.

4.09 pm
It's a longer wait today. I'm getting edgy.

4.27 pm
I'm finally checked in to the ward, and am sitting up on the bed in my hospital gown when a nurse comes by to complete the routine paperwork. She notes my tension and tells me to breathe. We fill in the questionnaire together. Any previous procedures? Yes, recent biopsy. Any medical conditions?

'Yes, cancer,' I say. I wonder why she didn't know, why that hadn't been communicated from one part of the hospital to another as the reason for my colonoscopy today.

'What type,' she asks.

I hate it when people ask me that. It feels like they're prying into my private business.

'Of the anal canal,' I answer, nevertheless.

'I'm so sorry,' she says.

Someone messages from the Facebook group. A complete stranger.

'Keep your eye on the horizon at all times,' she advises.

I love that image. I can see the horizon where the sky meets the sea in the distance from the back of my house. I'll take her advice and keep my eye firmly on it at least once each day.

Another Chatter, as group members are called, suggests I give my cancer a name. She called hers Colin. Mine will be Alan, I decide, an anagram of what it is. There you go. I'm getting a little more comfortable using the medical name of my cancerous body part. People still beat about the bush. The C word. That which shall not be named. Call it by its name. Naming makes it less unknown. Not so nice to meet you, Alan. I'm hoping our acquaintance will be short-lived.

Everything unknown is scary. My mother died from ovarian cancer at the age of 85. She was terrified of all things medical, all her life. She waited too long to seek help when cancer invaded her body and when she finally did it was too late. I hope I didn't leave mine too long. The doctors have told me that the size of the tumour indicates we got it in time.

Face it, name it, tame the beast. I can do hard things.

I have an uninvited guest in my body. I have cancer of the anal canal, otherwise known as Alan. He'll hang around for a while, it'll take some time and some pretty nasty treatment to get rid of him. But get rid of him I will.

5.23 pm

Time is dragging. What a job, looking up people's backsides. Doctors must be slightly crazy. Crazy but amazing.

5.45 pm

We're off. I'm wheeled into theatre. Joe the anaesthetist inspects my veins.

'They're tiny,' he says. I'm in Groundhog Day.

'I'll see if I can find one in your wrist.' Then, 'bullseye!' he says.

'Is it in?' I ask, once again thinking my un-woke thoughts.

'You sound surprised,' he says.

'They had trouble the other day,' I tell him.

'He's been doing this for a long time,' says the colonoscopy doctor, who's also in the room, waiting to probe my behind once the anaesthetic kicks in.

'Joe the pro,' I say, and chuckle at my own hilarity. They seem like friends, the doctor and the anaesthetist, a close team as they go about their business of inspecting backsides.

The day ends on a high. The colonoscopy is good, apart from a polyp, which is no more. The bowel preparation was excellent, says the report. I've always taken pride in a good report. I've got this.

Comment from Chat 10 Looks 3:
Take care, Sue. I love the strength and good humour you are showing already with the name Alan. You have thousands of Chatters backing you. x

30 March 2021
Horizon of hope

6.45 am
I sleep fitfully and worry about not getting back to sleep each time I wake, which only perpetuates the vicious cycle of insomnia. I heard on a podcast that insufficient sleep can make you more susceptible to cancer. Too late now.

When the alarm goes, I feel remarkably OK. As I wait for my coffee to brew, I stare at the morning sky, stretching to the horizon. I notice the moon, hanging just above the tree line. It's a full moon, I think. Ian pointed it out as we drove back from hospital last night and it's still there, sinking now, towards the horizon, my horizon of hope. It's so beautiful.

I feel love for all humankind after the deluge of virtual support sent yesterday, from complete strangers. I don't feel anger or self-pity or even sadness this morning. I feel strangely calm. I've got this. An online community across this great southern land are there for me. I'm aware of the dopamine hit from the surge of likes and emojis and affirming comments. It won't last, but I'll take it for now. I need all the help I can get.

Jess's concerns come into my mind again, for some reason. Her insistence that I be kind to myself. I'm good at giving myself the time and space to do the things that make my heart sing. I'm kind to myself in that way. It's to my mind that I'm not so kind. I can hold on to poisonous stuff for far too long, or revisit it more than is healthy.

'The feel of your photography and writing is so uplifting and expansive,' Jess told me when we spoke. I need to apply that same feeling to myself.

Expansive. Horizons. I like those words.

Later

Being back at work this morning seems surreal. Last night my insides were being probed under anaesthetic and now here I am teaching Year 8 French. I tell the class at the start of the lesson that I've been unwell and really need them to work quietly. Something in the way I speak conveys the message. They aren't the best listeners, 13-year-old boys, but they settle more quickly than usual.

When the bell goes, I commend them on their focus, adding that it was the most productive lesson of the term.

'Why do you think that was?' I ask.

'Because we listened, Miss, and concentrated,' says one.

'I got lots done,' says another.

'See what you can achieve when you put your mind to it,' I say, before wishing them a Happy Easter.

They head off, jostling and pushing their way through the door with boyish physicality, without a care in the world, thanking me for the lesson. Whatever their mood, behaviour or interest in learning on any given day, they always thank me for the lesson.

I'm leaving school early for a follow-up appointment with my surgeon, but not before I've told the Year 12s why I've been absent on and off for the last two weeks. I stick to the facts and reassure them that they'll be well looked after should I need more time off next term. I leave them in the library with our French assistant who will help them prepare for the speaking component of their exam next term. I've prepared work and instructions for them. They have plenty to do.

12.00 pm

Ian meets me at the hospital for the appointment. We sit a little anxiously, waiting to see the surgeon again to find out what the next step will be after the anal surgery and the colonoscopy.

I may be imagining things, but Charles seems less engaged than last week, more distant. Not quite as lovely. I guess this is routine for him, working through the process, but it's huge for me.

When he starts talking, my heart sinks as I try to process the information and realise just how many more hoops there are to jump through before Alan can be zapped. I'll need two different appointments next week to discuss chemotherapy and radiotherapy. My "team" – Charles, Greg, the radiotherapy oncologist and Simon, the chemotherapy oncologist – will then meet to coordinate my treatment plan, and I will need another scan at the radiotherapy clinic.

So far, so routine. But there's more. Charles tells me the PET scan showed a "hot spot" somewhere around my throat and neck, which the team feels warrants further investigation with an ENT specialist. He gives me the name of the doctor he would like me to see – Dr Tony somebody – and tells me his receptionist will contact the ENT receptionist to make (yet another) appointment.

'This won't affect the cancer treatment,' he adds, looking down at his notes.

Now I understand the reason for his more distant manner – he knew he had to deliver some unexpected news.

'What the fuck?' I silently mouth, glancing nervously at Ian, who shrugs helplessly and takes my hand, which helps, while also grimacing and widening his eyes in alarm, which doesn't help.

It's more than alarming, a setback I hadn't anticipated. I'm unsure what a "hot spot" means and wonder why it wasn't mentioned after surgery, when Charles came to reassure me that the biopsy had gone smoothly and the cancer hadn't spread.

He explains that it's a mild something or other (I can't remember the exact word), not necessarily a tumour, but it's an added worry when I thought all was clear. All clear apart from Alan, that is. When I ask questions to try to establish a timeframe, Charles tells me I should hear within a week or so, which all sounds a bit vague. He tries to reassure me, and says that if I haven't heard anything in the next couple of weeks I could call the ENT rooms myself to follow up. The baton is being passed on. I must be patient. But I'm confused and agitated by this new development. There'll now be a fourth member of my specialist team.

Charles is due in theatre, to probe some other Alans no doubt, and leaves us with his receptionist. She tries to contact both oncology doctors to help me set up the treatment planning appointments. I feel like I'm swimming against an unstoppable tide, drowning in a tsunami of appointments and scans and phone calls and follow-ups. There's so much to coordinate, and I'm grateful for the receptionist's kind assistance. We wait. Eventually contact is made with one but the other isn't answering. They should call you tomorrow, she says.

More waiting.

8.00 pm

I fit in a walk later, and do some yoga poses, and it feels good. Contrary to the advice given by a nurse last week, Charles told me earlier today that there's no problem with either swimming in the ocean, or doing moderate weights or any form of exercise, in fact. Thank god. That was one positive to come out of this morning's appointment. A kind of medical shit sandwich, I now think, chuckling despite myself: you can walk every day, you have a hot spot that warrants further investigation, you can swim in the ocean.

I'm grateful for the much-needed outlet, for the physical and mental release that comes with moving my body, thankful that I can do whatever I'm comfortable doing and continue with my normal life.

Normal life? Will my life ever be normal again?

I'm tired now. Very tired. I don't think I've fully processed that I'll be having chemotherapy soon. I do some lesson preparation for tomorrow. It feels good to do something that I can control when I can't control any of this medical process. I know I must have faith in the doctors, trust that things will keep moving and that the oncologist will call tomorrow. Another step, another hoop. Line them up and keep on jumping.

Comment from Chat 10 Looks 3 Community:
We are so fortunate to live in the lucky country. Top class medical care. Place your trust in your health professionals and take it all one day at a time. Never be afraid to ask questions. Good luck with everything.

31 March 2021

Enough

A new month beckons, a fresh perspective. On any given day I will deal with Alan in a different way. On some days I'll draw strength from messages and emails and online support. On others I'll need to get off my phone and out of my head. Sometimes I'll need silence and space. Sometimes I'll need company and laughter. There is no right or wrong way to get through this. The right way, is, I guess, to do what comes naturally, to not put pressure on myself to be a certain type of cancer patient. *I can only be me.*

The Chat 10 Looks 3 community continues to rally around, sending love, advice and support. Everyone wants to help. People are so nice. Complete strangers tell me things that make me cry, just because they stopped what they were doing and took the time to convey their concern. The name Alan has been greeted with much hilarity.

'Great name (insert crying with laughter emoji),' someone writes.

'Death to Alan,' adds another.

'I once knew an Alan, and he was an arsehole,' writes someone else.

'What a bummer' and 'Get fucked Alan,' write plenty more.

I've skipped a day of writing, but that's OK. I went to work yesterday and taught all day. By 3.30 pm I was drained. That's it, I thought. Enough.

At the start of the day, as I ticked off the names of the boys in my House tutor group, and they collected their school photos, a colleague asked how my term had been. He obviously hadn't been in Monday's briefing meeting, when my news was announced to staff. I put him in the picture, as gently as I could. He was so sorry. He told me he wouldn't be coming to school if he were in my situation.

'You're very committed,' he said.

Committed or foolish, I think later. Time to put my health first. Between classes I met with the HR manager once again. The message remains consistent. *Put yourself first. Don't worry about work. Your job is secure. Take all the leave you need. We'll work it out.*

I told him I was tired and would take tomorrow off. Then it will be Easter, and a two-week break.

'No problem,' he said.

There are parent teacher interviews all day, from which I've been excused, and I only have one class to teach. It can be easily covered.

When I left the HR office, I sat down in the staff room to gather myself. A colleague walked in, looking flustered, a huge pile of marking under his arm. I asked how he was.

'Not good,' he said. 'So much to do.'

He then asked about my plans for the holidays. He clearly hadn't heard my news either.

I take a breath and tell him I'll be starting cancer treatment. He looks taken aback. Why do I feel uncomfortable? Why do I feel the urge to then apologise for answering his question? I tell myself not to feel awkward. This is real. This is life. This is what I will be doing in the holidays.

When I tell Ian and Ben this anecdote later they think it's hilarious, and suggest it would make a great comedy sketch. We do some family improvisation of people saying the wrong thing, of putting their foot in it, of elephant-in-the-room scenarios. It's good to laugh, despite the blackness of our humour. I haven't had a really good laugh in a long time.

A few years ago, I attended a comedy masterclass in Melbourne. It was organised by the same woman who ran the self-publishing workshop I signed up for when writing my way out of depression. I had the time, I could stay with Marita, why not?

It was terrifying. At the end of the day, we had to deliver a three-minute stand-up routine, without notes. Somehow, I got through, babbling on about hot yoga, the inability of WA drivers to merge, and other hard-hitting comedic gems. People laughed. It felt good. I like to make people laugh. And boy do I have some material now that Alan has come into my life. My *anus horribilis*. Killing Alan. Putting cancer behind me.

I digress. The headmaster emails again, offering his support.

'Is there anything we can do?' he writes. 'If you're comfortable, I could send an email to all staff,' he offers, telling me that if I touch base with his PA, she will organise it.

I take him up on his offer and go through the wording with her. When I briefly lose it and the tears flow, she's calm and kind and once again I feel deeply grateful for the school community.

Two more classes to go after lunch. I've put all that I can in place to help my students prepare for exams. Time to let go, for a while.

Yesterday I told my Year 12s the news. Today I tell my Year 11s. They listen and take it all in their stride. They are refreshingly accepting. I feel completely comfortable. One boy asks what type of cancer I have. I tell him I'm not going to discuss that and gently ask him to respect my wishes. Some of the others show exasperation with their classmate with tutting and eye rolls. They get it. His question was insensitive, not appropriate. But he's a child and he's curious. I don't mind.

Another student asks, 'RU OK, Miss?'

I nearly lose it, then smile and tell him that yes, I'm as OK as I can be, I'm happy to be here at this great school, I'm glad to be here teaching you.

We get on with the lesson, discuss exams and orals and revision, chat about sport towards the end. Some of them know Ben, through hockey and cricket, and often ask about him, probably to distract me from teaching them convoluted grammatical rules such as the agreement of the past participle with the preceding direct object. I realise this, of course, I'm fully aware of such distraction strategies. I didn't come down in the last shower, as my mother would say.

But, in spite of their teenage tactics, I sense they do have a genuine interest in my son, and I like these connections. When the lesson ends, I tell them I'll see them next term sometime, but I'm not sure when. They wish me well and are gone.

I sit in the stillness of my empty classroom for a while, focussing on my breath, feeling my heartbeat. Life continues.

Comment from Chat 10 Looks 3 Community:
All the biggest gentle hugs to you. It's such a tough road but we are lucky to live in a country where medical care is so good and available. Reach out to us anytime.

1 April 2021
Eye on the horizon

A dose of cleansing salt water and sea-spray scented air this morning to soothe the soul. I walk on the beach for an hour or so, dipping in and out of the ocean to cool off when I need to. It's hot today.

I sit for a while afterwards and listen to the waves, gazing out to sea. A few fishermen dot the shoreline. Dog walkers pass. The horizon, my horizon of hope, is a precision-cut line in the distance.

Back home I message some friends, chat to another, make some lunch, do a sudoku.

I lie down for a rest. Ben comes home from work. Some flowers arrive at the door. Ian returns. The school holidays begin.

Comment from Chat 10 Looks 3 Community:
It must be so hard for you not to have your son nearby as you go through this. Be kind to yourself, accept help offered and ask for help too. Meditation and positive imagery helped me. Sending love, hugs and healing thoughts to you.

2 April 2021, Good Friday
Winning deep

9.30 am
Last night I had my first social outing since Alan came into my life. Ben's hockey fixture was at home, a short walk across the fields from our house. Earlier, I'd messaged some friends I expected to see there to tell them my news. It would help if a few people knew in advance, I thought. Saves explaining it all again and again, as with my flustered colleague on Wednesday.

The team was just finishing their warm-up when I arrived. Ian followed on his bike after a gym workout. Ben was playing premier league, then doubling up with the second team, as several players always do.

A friend approached and gave me a big hug.

'Ian told me your news,' he said. My eyes well up.

'You'll make me cry,' I told him.

We stood for a while, arm in arm, not needing to talk much. He's been through his own variety of Alan. A couple of times, in fact. And lived to tell both tales. He'll be cheering for me, all the way.

His wife joined us and we sat to watch the game. I put my arm through hers and my head on her shoulder briefly and told her it's nice to see her, good to do something normal. The club was buzzing with anticipation, spectators eating and drinking and celebrating the start of the Easter weekend. It was still hot. The game started, a clash of fierce rivals, the opposition coached by Australian hockey legend Ric Charlesworth.

Ben looked comfortable on the field and played well in a fast-paced, end-to-end match. Normally I react to every move and cheer the team on, but last night I just sat and observed and didn't get too concerned when the opposition took the lead. Ben's team played catch-up and couldn't quite get there, despite a late goal.

Between quarters I talked to a few more friends I'd texted earlier. Two of them stood either side of me and the three of us put our arms around each other. One kissed me firmly on the cheek, squeezing me tighter, and we stayed like that for a while, not saying anything at all.

When the first game ended and the second warm-up started, I chatted with Jacky, another hockey friend. I don't know her well, but we've always had a nice rapport. She's an oncology nurse at a big public hospital. We often see each other at the beach. She'll run past me at four times my walking speed and come back again before I've reached the point where I turn around.

Now, at the hockey club, she hugged me tight when I took a deep breath and told her my news.

'I knew something was wrong when I saw you at the beach the other day,' she said. 'I could sense it.'

She's in the business, so to speak. Her cancer radar must be highly developed.

We chatted about Alan and she asked which oncologists would be overseeing my chemotherapy and radiotherapy. I checked their names on my phone. She knows them well. They're lovely, apparently. At the top of their game and great with patients, which is comforting to know. She lives around the corner from me and will keep in touch.

I asked her advice about taking leave from work, wondering if a term might be enough, depending on the length of treatment required, which I'll find out next week. Jacky urged me to take at least two terms off.

'You'll need time to recover once treatment ends, Sue. You need to focus on yourself,' she said. 'I advise all my patients to take at least six months off. Your body has given you a message. You need to heed it. You need to slow down.'

When I was at school, I was what would today be called a high achiever. My parents expected nothing less. I won a school prize every year, except for one, but we didn't talk about that. I was a straight-A student, except in science, but we didn't talk about that. I made the 1st XI hockey team when I was 15, we won the Northern Irish schools' cup, were featured on the local television news and attended a dinner at the town hall to celebrate the victory. We talked about that a lot.

I also played first team tennis and won the school tennis cup in consecutive years. And, to crown it all, I won the school table tennis trophy (yes, we really had a table tennis trophy) at least once, if not twice.

I played first clarinet in the school orchestra after debuting early as second clarinettist. I performed clarinet solos and piano duets at school concerts. I sang in the school choir and performed in a few drama productions. No lead roles, though, apart from the last year of primary school when I played a poor servant girl who tears a princess's ball dress and embarks on an against-the-clock quest to mend the delicate fabric. She succeeds, with the help of a wise old woman and some magical tailors, I seem to remember. I feel like I need a wise old woman and some magic right now.

Despite all this, I was painfully shy, terrified of my teachers, fearful of public speaking and had little or no self-esteem (I didn't even know self-esteem was a thing). If we'd had any geese, I wouldn't have said boo to them. I knew a lot of facts and could do a lot of things, but I didn't receive a rounded education. I didn't receive an education that prepared me for life.

I'd give it all back, the A grades and the medals and trophies, all of it in a heartbeat, if I could rewind and emerge from school as a self-aware, self-confident, self-accepting, complete person.

When we first came to Perth, I started playing serious hockey again. There's a long-standing tradition of hockey in Western Australia, excellent facilities, strong competitions. The men's and women's national teams are based in Perth. Ben and Daniel used to watch me from the sidelines when they were little, until my knees and ankles could take it no more.

Hockey is a great team game. I love the fact that I passed the baton (or should I say the stick) on to the boys. Ian played too, as did his father and my father, so it's in our genes. Daniel doesn't play anymore, now that he lives overseas. He was a very talented junior (one coach named him The Wizard due to his magical stick skills), but competition wasn't his thing. He didn't love it enough. Now I see that the expectation to compete and win took all the fun out of sport for him. We play sport, but rarely embrace the spirit of playfulness.

In the second act of my hockey career, I pushed myself to the limit, and beyond. Too far, too much. I played for the over-40s state team in the early 2000s. At the National Championships one year I rolled my ankle so badly in a key match I had to crawl off the pitch in agony. The physiotherapist got to work and strapped me up. I missed one game and then was back. We made it to the semi-finals and came third.

For three months afterwards I could barely walk.

A couple of days ago I listened to Dr Pippa Grange on Brené Brown's *Dare to Lead* podcast. Pippa is a highly sought-after sports psychologist, recognised as the person who helped break the England football team's penalty shoot-out curse in the 2018 World Cup. She talked about the need to be a soulful and wholehearted competitor, whatever level you are playing at, or whatever you are doing in life. She told several anecdotes in which I recognised myself, and it wasn't comfortable.

She spoke of open hearts versus clenched fists. I thought I was an open-hearted person, but I know those clenched fists well. The two doctors, Brown and Grange, discussed fear, anxiety and perfectionism. I recognised myself time and time again in their conversation.

Pippa has written a book (of course she has): *Fear Less: How to Win at Life Without Losing Yourself.* I need to read it. I downloaded a sample on my Kindle but want to buy the hard copy so I can highlight and underline and re-read passages. In Chapter Two, she writes about "winning shallow", which leaves you unsatisfied and wanting more, moving quickly from one so called achievement to the next, as opposed to "winning deep". Have I ever won deep, I wonder?

I'm tired now. I don't feel able to do anything much. It's exactly two weeks since I found out I have anal cancer. This is the first day since my diagnosis that I've not been thinking about work, or appointments, or how to fit everything into the day. It's a strange feeling. I start to let go. Tired is an understatement. I'm mentally exhausted, wiped out.

I lie on the bed and flick through some TV channels before settling on an ABC documentary about Easter. I've never understood why the dates of Easter are different each year. It's something to do with the first full moon and the Spring equinox,

I hear an earnest religious leader explain, but I still don't really understand. My eyelids start to flutter. I'm moving in and out of slumber. I give in and drift away.

Comment from Chat 10 Looks 3 Community:
Thinking of you, Sue. You are not alone on this journey. Take care.

3 April 2021
Surrender

Yesterday, I surrendered (how apt, I now think, to do so on the day that Christ was crucified). As the Easter documentary rolled, my body and mind shut down. Each time I resurfaced I found I could barely move. Every muscle ached. I stumbled to the kitchen on jelly-weak legs to make tea and fruit toast, then staggered straight back to bed. I stayed put and gave myself over to whatever universal forces were at play.

Hours later, I re-emerged to some form of consciousness feeling ravenous and had some more to eat. I then decamped to the front room and reclined once more to watch an undemanding romantic movie on Amazon Prime, set in Bruges. Total frippery, the plotline predictable, but it was nice to look at and I enjoyed it.

I went to Bruges once, in 1982, with the family of one of my students, when I was a French teaching assistant in the north of France. I probably didn't fully appreciate its beauty back then. From the comfort of the sofa I called out to Ian to tell him we have to put Bruges on our list. I want to go back.

Ian came to join me and, as he stroked my aching legs, told me we will indeed go to Bruges. He'd just been shopping for essentials and things he knows I like – yoghurt, avocado, raspberries, bananas.

Feeling a little restored after the film, I made us a chicken and avocado salad, adding fresh basil and Ben's homemade dressing. Delicious. I then settled down once more to watch another movie. The last time I watched movies back-to-back was on a plane.

'Imagine you are on a long-haul flight in first class,' Ian joked.

We both miss travel so much. As I watched, Ian kept coming in and out of the room, checking to see if I was comfortable, if I needed anything, to rub my shoulders and hold me close. He's so thoughtful, this man of mine.

The second film was set in rural England. The countryside was picture perfect. A former top chef, grieving for his wife, buys the old pub they had planned to renovate together before she died. He rediscovers his culinary flair, of course, is feted by the critics, of course, and finds romance once more, of course, but not before the requisite conflicts are dealt with and resolved. Nice.

As the credits rolled, Ian offered to drive me to the beach to watch the sunset.

'I'd love that,' I told him.

We arrived at the perfect moment and bathed in an ocean of liquid gold, then sat in the dunes to gaze at the horizon until the last glow of orange has left the sky.

It was dark when we got home. I felt like a walk, and headed off into the night, headphones on, to walk and talk to my friend Sarah, sticking to well-lit roads. I updated her on the past week. She agreed about work and urged me to give myself time, to put myself first.

Sarah has progressive MS and depends on her wheelchair and the care of her wonderful husband, Sammy. She's one of the most positive people I know. She lives in a little town in Northern

Ireland, near where we both grew up. Sarah is my oldest friend, not in terms of age but in years of friendship.

'I did well today,' I told her. 'I listened to my body and stayed horizontal for most of the day.'

Sarah approved. She knows of my high-achieving urges.

'And how are you?' I asked.

She looked great. Her hair is white now, but her face is youthful, unlined, unchanged. We were on video chat, and as I looked at the screen she told me not to fall over in the dark, to watch my step. She could see the cars passing. I held the phone down and switched to audio mode so I could focus on the path. For a fleeting moment I wondered if there was more risk of me being hit by a car while out walking than the worst-case Alan scenario.

The thought of speeding cars reminded me that on the day after my biopsy, a woman knocked on my door to tell me she'd broken a sprinkler on our verge. She was sorry and would, of course, pay for it. She wrote down her details and I thanked her for her honesty.

'Not everyone would do this,' I told her.

Soon afterwards, my neighbour, Cathy, messaged to say she had stopped a woman in a huge SUV who had sped down our road and used our driveway to do a U turn while crunching over our sprinkler, oblivious to the breakage. Cathy apprehended her, just as she was driving off, pointing out what she had done and urging her to own up and let me, the owner of the damaged sprinkler, know.

'Did she contact you,' Cathy messages.

'She did indeed,' I tell her. 'Thanks to you.'

Not so honest, then, my sprinkler damaging friend. More like shamed into confession. Ian organised the sprinkler repair, sent the invoice, and she paid forthwith.

It's a random anecdote, I realise, in the context of my situation, but how much damage do we cause, I wonder, by not paying attention? We all need to pay more attention. Why was the woman speeding in a school zone? Why did she feel the need to do a U turn instead of using the roundabout less than 100 metres further down the road? Rush, rush, rush, the adult ADHD of our times.

Yesterday I paid attention to my body, and it felt good. I took my time, and it felt good. I stopped fretting, and it felt good. I ate what I wanted, when I was hungry, and it felt good. I rested for most of the day, and it felt good.

After my walk, I found a few more messages. One from a colleague wishing me well for the break and telling me everyone is thinking of me. Another from a former colleague, someone I haven't seen for years, sending me love and light. She's heard my news on the grapevine. I'm comfortable with people knowing, for news to trickle through in due course. I don't want to hide it or lock it away like some shameful secret.

Back to the present. I had resolved to do more of the same today, to spend most of it lying down, but I'm feeling stronger than yesterday. Strong enough to do a little gentle exercise this morning. A few yoga poses, some stretches and abdominals. It feels comfortable, eases my worry for a while. I take my time, listening to music and lying still on my mat for a while afterwards.

Ian leaves for the day, to visit his parents, but not before shopping for Easter eggs for tomorrow. Ben recently enquired about the traditional family egg hunt. We were non-committal.

'Maybe not this year,' we said.

But the Easter Bunny will oblige after all. Ever thoughtful, my husband. Life goes on, we must have eggs and they must be hunted. While at the shops, he sees some headlines for articles in *The Australian* he thinks I'd like. Far more satisfying than the digital version but an endangered species, no doubt, an actual newspaper, a broadsheet, no less. I'll enjoy it while it lasts.

I make a hearty brunch of scrambled eggs, avocado, tomato mushrooms and devour it while reading of comedian Judith Lucy's discovery that she's OK after all and learning about all things "woke" among other news and features. It almost feels like a normal Saturday.

When I was growing up, I loved Easter, perhaps more than Christmas. I believed in the magic long after my rational mind knew it could not be so. I cherished the collection of enticingly packaged, foil-wrapped eggs that appeared each Easter Sunday morning. I would count them again and again, calculate how many days I could make them last, arrange them in colourful clusters of jewel-like splendour.

I try to remember the last time we were all together for Easter, our family foursome. When the boys were little, the egg hunt was a highlight, their shiny eyes growing larger as they filled their baskets. I suddenly feel terribly sad as I remember those uncomplicated days before COVID separated us.

6 April 2021
Reality bites

7.17 am
Easter has been and gone and it starts to get real again today. After nearly a week of waiting, in a couple of hours I have an appointment to discuss chemotherapy. I guess they have to talk you through everything, make sure you understand the side-effects and so on. I don't want to do all that. Just hook me up and start pumping the stuff through my sick body. My mind has been

imagining all sorts of horrors this last week, all manner of grim scenarios. I need to get out of my mind and focus on my body.

Georgia recommended a book when we spoke on Easter Sunday: *Chatter*, by neuroscientist and psychologist, Ethan Kross. I've downloaded a sample on my Kindle to try before I buy.

According to the blurb, Kross has spent his entire professional life researching the conversations we have with ourselves, what they are, why we have them and how they can be harnessed to make us "happier, healthier and more productive". Who doesn't want that? Post-Alan – yes, there will be a post-Alan I keep telling myself – perhaps he can help me become a newly happy, healthy and productive me.

You'd think that with all the experts who've written books about the human condition we'd have it sorted out by now and be living our best lives. So many self-help books, each claiming to possess the magic formula for enlightenment, for an unencumbered life. I've read more than a few in my time. Shouldn't we only ever need to read one? Shouldn't such books, by definition, if they do what they claim on the cover, help you help yourself, find yourself, be your best self, to the extent that you never need to read another one of them?

I talked to Georgia for an hour or so at the end of a quiet Easter Sunday. There was no lavish celebration in our house. Ben worked all morning in the café before hunting for and finding his eggs. Ian and I watched a French movie in the city, stopped off at the beach for another splendid sunset, came home, ate dinner, watched something on iView. Then Georgia called.

At the sound of her voice, I started to sob.

'I don't know if I can talk,' I said. 'I'm so tired, and sad.'

And so scared, I realised, so very scared.

Some people don't know how to react when someone is upset. Some people always manage to make it all about them and the experiences they've had or tell you about friends who've been through this, that and the other. Who cut you off before you've finished what you want to say. Who constantly interrupt. Or tell you to stop crying, it isn't so bad. Or remind you how much you have to be grateful for. Or tell you there are many far worse off than you.

Comparative suffering, it's so unhealthy, so shaming. No one was ever shamed into feeling better. On the contrary. Just ask Brené Brown.

Georgia isn't one of those people. She's easy to talk to, endlessly kind and patient, a great listener. Her background as a journalist could be something to do with it.

I remember reading, years ago, about an approach to trauma called the SUMO method. It works, said the author of the piece, with what I felt was limited awareness of the human condition. SUMO, in this case, is not a Japanese martial art. It stands for Shut Up Move On. At the time, I was trying to process all kinds of family baggage and failing miserably. I was overwhelmed and anxious, drowning in grief, spiralling into depression. The last thing I needed to do was Shut Up. I needed to let it all out before I could even begin to Move On.

I didn't take the SUMO advice. Instead, I wrote a book. It worked, to a large extent. I moved on with my life, came to realise that the family baggage would always be there, but that I could choose whether to carry it or not. With time, I managed to shrink the baggage to the size of a small carry-on case. Occasionally, a piece of hold luggage reappears to torment me, urging me to lift it off the airport conveyor belt until, with an immense force of will, I tell myself it belongs to someone else.

Now that I'm in the middle of another health crisis I can't help wishing I could confide in my siblings, knowing that whatever I said I'd be buoyed by a sea of love, compassion and understanding.

I'm an idiot, I know. My own worst enemy. I still haven't told my brother and sister about Alan, and I still don't know what to do about that. I'm scared, most likely irrationally so, about what they might say about him. About me.

They say that friends are the family we choose for ourselves. And it's true. My friends feel like family. But those goddamn blood ties, they've come back to haunt me just when I least need to be haunted. The friends I've told about Alan will buoy me, scoop me up and carry me through. Ian tells me there's no reason why my siblings wouldn't do the same. He's knows it's complicated and hard after so much grief and loss and things said and not said and all that family stuff.

Last night, two friends did a bit of scooping and took me out for a pizza and a glass of wine and it felt so good. There was just enough chat about the medical side of things, and then it was on to our kids and husbands and holidays and work, which is just how I want it to be. The balance was perfect. No awkward ignoring of the awfulness of cancer, no beating around any bushes, but no dwelling on the negative. Cheers to those two women.

On Sunday night, as I tried to talk between sobs, Georgia listened attentively, somehow finding the right words at the right time. My weeping subsided and the conversation moved on. She has finally "completed" on her new London flat. That's the English way. You exchange contracts and then you complete. She hasn't moved in but has the keys. There's still a bit to do. I'm excited for her. She has plans for the kitchen and bathroom, hopes to install some French doors leading onto the little garden. I can't wait to be there and sleep in what she calls "Sue's room".

It was late when we finished talking. Way past my bedtime. My tears had dried, for now. I curled up with my Kindle and drifted in and out of slumber, taking refuge from the dialogue running through my head, if only for a while.

Comment from Chat 10 Looks 3 Community:
Some people just cannot deal with what is happening to you ... and react in weird and unhelpful ways. Sometimes support comes when you least expect it and not necessarily from those closest to you.

7 April 2021
I don't want to talk about it

Ian has taken to watching clips on YouTube of the inside of aeroplanes. He loves everything about planes and flying and wishes he could have been a pilot. As a child, he once went into the cockpit of a Boeing 747 and remembers the thrill of drawing back the curtain, which was all that divided the pilot from the passengers in those days, and stepping into a wonderland of lights and control panels. He was enchanted to find himself in the driving seat of his dreams. Each time we board a plane that magic returns for Ian. He's like a kid in a candy store.

While scrolling mindlessly on my phone, I see some posts about Tasmania. I really want to go there, and to New Zealand.

'We must go when all this is over,' I tell Ian. 'There is so much still to do, so many places I want to see.'

He agrees.

'We'll get there,' he says.

I've tried to stay busy over the last few days, keeping up with exercise and going for walks. I'm fed up with Alan. I want him gone. I'm so tired. I don't know if it's mental or physical fatigue, or both. I spent Monday morning at the beach, reading, walking and swimming. In the afternoon Ian came with me to another

French film, which we both found a little laboured and clunky. I so wanted to escape for another two hours but was fidgety and restless as I waited for it to end.

Yesterday I met Simon, my chemotherapy oncologist, for the first time. He seems lovely and was as reassuring as he could be in the circumstances. My overactive mind doesn't like to hear about percentages and potential complications and risk factors, about less than ideal outcomes, but he has to tell it like it is. The next step is to see the radiotherapy oncologist this afternoon. Then both oncologists will liaise before l find out my starting date. I hope the wait won't be too long. I asked Simon if I can go down south in the meantime and he encouraged me to do just that, to get away, take my mind off all of this, carry on as normal.

Normal? What's that, I ask myself again.

While I'm at the radiotherapy clinic, Ian will drive out to the airport to pick up his other sister, Jane. It's their Dad's 80th tomorrow. Both sisters will cross over for a couple of days before Anne flies back to Sydney on Friday. I don't feel up to the planned celebratory lunch. Celebration, what celebration? My father-in-law in a wheelchair and me with cancer. It may be his last birthday, but no one says it. I find it all unbearably sad. He may surprise us all, though, and live to the age of 100, as did his mother.

I drive to the clinic as if on autopilot. I'll be doing this trip every day for six weeks once treatment starts. The glum weather mirrors my mood. Layers of cloud hang resolutely overhead on a grey-sky day. They ain't going nowhere, those clouds, not today.

The clinic is modern, open plan, clean and bright. The staff are friendly and welcoming. I see the oncologist on time. He starts with an internal examination. A nurse holds my hand while he puts his up my backside. Lovely. Probing over, he explains the process of radiation and what it aims to achieve. He is calm and patient and tells me the facts, sparing no detail. I don't want to hear it all, chapter and verse, I'm not keen on listening to worst-case scenarios, but he's duty bound to tell me. It's a lot to take in.

Ian arrives towards the end of the appointment, after the airport pick-up. I can't decide whether I want him there or not. Sometimes I just want to be on my own. I don't want him asking questions for me, questions to which I don't necessarily want to know the answers. But then again, walking this path truly alone would be unbearable I imagine.

Fate intervenes when my planning and CT scan appointment is scheduled for tomorrow. The only remaining slot this week clashes with the birthday lunch. I have to take it. Am I selfish for feeling relieved I don't have to front up to a family lunch? I have to take the appointment and keep this ball rolling. Maybe it's for the best; I wouldn't be much company and Ian's Dad will enjoy having his three children together for the day.

Ian goes straight home from the clinic, but I head to the beach to forget for a while. I walk and swim and listen to music, inhaling the sea air deeply, willing it to soothe me, to nourish and heal my broken body.

It's dark when I get home. Jane is full of chat and questions when I really don't want to talk about anything medical, about procedures and treatment schedules and prognoses. Her hair is cancer-short, a reminder of what may lie ahead for me. Her breast cancer surgery and treatment have worked well. She clutches her "new boob", showing me that she's a survivor and proud of it, and so she should be.

But when she starts to ask about my treatment, I tell her I'm not up to a discussion at the moment. I try to explain, as politely as I can, that I don't want to talk about it, and then feel bad about doing so. I'm irritated and uneasy. Jane is a guest in my house, she's curious and wants to help, but her questions feel intrusive.

Other people's curiosity is not more important that my comfort and well-being. At least that's what I try to tell myself, without much success. Jane is a kind person and wants nothing but the best for me.

It's such a minefield, this friends and family and help and support stuff. Of course, I need support, I need all the support I can get, but sometimes I just need silence and acceptance, not chatter and questions. A friend called a couple of days ago, a friend whose husband didn't win his cancer battle. It was less than a year ago, and yet she still takes the time to check in with me. We talked about how to navigate queries and questions and she told me that sometimes it all got too overwhelming for them, especially towards the end when they just wanted to bed down as a family. She tells me I absolutely must put myself first.

There's no right or wrong way to be, I realise. You are how you are on any given day. It is what it is. I mustn't beat myself up if I can't be how other people want me to be. Their comfort is not more important than my reality.

Tonight, I'm tired and irritable and I just want to lose myself in some easy viewing at the end of the day rather than field medical questions I don't want to answer.

I try, and fail, to shake off my resentment. Jane is keen to offer advice and talk through the treatment with me, but that's not what I need right now. Ben looks uncomfortable. He knows his aunt means well but I feel the plot has not been read. I wish people understood that everyone deals with cancer in different ways, that they do not have the right to invade my need to shield myself from their curiosity, no matter how well intended.

We have dinner, tidy up, watch *Hard Quiz*, wind down, prepare for the night. I've downloaded some podcasts and have a new book on my Kindle for nocturnal entertainment should sleep evade me.

Comment from Chat 10 Looks 3 Cancer Consortium:
The "Good Vibes Only" crowd are, somewhat paradoxically, such a downer. Maybe try 'thanks, but I'm not looking for advice, just a listening ear.'

8 April 2021
Escape

I slept on and off again. I wish I could crack the secret code to getting a good night's sleep on a regular basis. I once met a sleep specialist at a party. It's an actual job, sleep specialist. Who knew? We bonded over margaritas and tales of woe about our unfortunately wired body clocks and I discovered that not being a morning person is a genuine thing. I am not lazy; I am just wired this way.

As for my frequent night-time waking, well, I learnt that this is also a thing; it's called sleep maintenance insomnia. I have no trouble getting to sleep but often wake up, seemingly for no reason at all, in the wee small hours. Now that I have Alan to contend with, my propensity to wake up several times during the night can unleash all kinds of disturbing thoughts.

When I stirred, I was too tired to focus on words on a page, but the podcasts got me through the periods of wakefulness. I like listening to experts from completely different fields, learning from people with ideas, experiences and perspectives totally different to my own. That's how we evolve and grow, not by having our quite possibly erroneous standpoints endorsed by the ever-decreasing narrowness of the Facebook/Instagram bubble.

Ah, Facebook and Instagram. Where would we be without them? A lot damn happier, I'm willing to bet. It seems that if you aren't on the cyber bandwagon of life you barely exist, can most certainly not "make a difference" and are definitely not a person worth knowing. If you don't have an online profile and a loyal following in the millions, then who the hell are you? I am followed, therefore I am.

I've made some half-hearted attempts to join in with the cyberchat and posting and story-telling and reeling but I'm terrible at Faceboasting and Instabragging. I like to post photographs of nature and small moments that give me joy, but that's about it. I clearly don't have the hashtag knowhow required to garner a vast following and even if I had a following, I don't know what I would do with it. Sell more books, I guess. Get more traffic to my website, according to Fred. That's why you post, he tells me. To gain followers, who might become readers, who would help me earn more than the pittance Amazon sends me every time I sell a book. Business acumen was never my forte.

Now that I'm writing about Alan, I wonder whether I could or should do some Insta-oversharing about my battle with cancer. To what avail? I don't have the stomach for it. The Chat 10 post I did was enough, for the time being. I'm not ready to share my vulnerability with the world just yet.

So, for now I'll keep writing this journal to process my thoughts as I walk this path and fight my battle, a battle that continues today as I drive to the radiotherapy clinic for my planning and scanning meeting.

The appointment is bang on time and all goes well. A nurse talks me through the treatment process again before I empty and then refill my bladder in preparation for the CT scan. The scan will ascertain the position of everything and ensure that the radiotherapy is directed to exactly the right place. There's a short wait before I'm taken to the scanning room, where I remove my underwear and lie flat and still, face up, under the machine. There are two clinic staff with me all the time – I'm not sure of their job title; they're not doctors or nurses, but their role in my treatment is vital. I'm positioned and then tattooed with three small dots to mark the target zone across the top of my pelvic bone. I'm adjusted and repositioned a little more (we're talking fractions of millimetres), the machine does its thing, and that's it. I'm good to go until treatment starts in 10 days.

I drive south to escape for a while, as planned. Ian will follow in a few days, when his sisters have swapped roles and he feels he can leave his parents in Jane's hands for a while. I'll find sanctuary "down south", in the corner of Western Australia that's one of my favourite places on Earth. After three weeks of back and forward to the hospital, and these last three days of intense appointments, I'm drained and depleted. I need peace and silence and space to just be.

9 April 2021
Respite

I sink into bed and sleep long and late. Do some exercise. Read for hours. Cycle to the swimming beach. Swim in the seaweed strewn bay. Cycle back. Go for a walk. Watch Graham Norton. Go to bed. Read some more. *I will be well, I will be well, I will be well.*

10 April 2021
Family matters

I sleep soundly again – the sleep specialist would be proud – but wake up with an aching neck, stiff shoulders and a tense upper back. I get up slowly and ease into the day, trying to unknot the tension in my upper body with some gentle stretching. A walk into town, a quick chat to Ian, some more stretching and exercise. The tension remains.

Anne calls. She's back in Sydney, having handed the family baton to Jane for the next week or so. Anne and I have been messaging over the last few days. She's the proverbial tower of strength. Every family has one, and Anne is ours. She tells me I must believe and have faith, that I must say out loud that I will be well again. She speaks with total conviction rather than offering lame platitudes. She's a rock and she's right. I need to make myself say it more often. I will be well. *The treatment will work. I've got this.*

Later, I walk and talk to Ian. It's an emotional conversation. The last couple of weeks have taken their toll. Our world has been turned upside down. We talk about his parents' situation and the way forward. Anne has done so much to set up extra help through government services and now we must wait to see if they deliver. It's a protracted process just to get an initial assessment organised and, even then, it can take up to a year for the help to be put in place. It seems absurd and wrong that fragile old people have such a long waiting period before help materialises. They could be dead by then. We've been told that, while they wait for the full care package to be set up, Ian's parents should start getting interim help by the time Jane has to leave, but it all sounds so piecemeal and unsatisfactory.

We talk about Ben. He's struggled with my news, Ian says. Ben hasn't said much to me, but he and Ian have been chatting in my absence and it's clear his world has been rocked. He wants to help me, Ian says, but doesn't always know what to do. I need to talk to him and tell him he just needs to be himself and walk beside me. He doesn't need to do anything special.

'I'm finding it so hard, this invasion of my body,' I tell Ian.

He understands but often feels helpless.

'How would you deal with it?' I ask him.

He tells me he would try to take every minute as it comes, and not think ahead too much. Focus on the here and now.

'That's easier said than done,' I say. 'Especially with a mind like mine.'

'Try to take your mind to good places,' he says. 'Don't let Alan infect your mind as well as your body.'

He's right, of course. I know all of this.

'I'll try to take control of my thoughts,' I tell him. 'I'm doing my best. I will get better. We will get to Tasmania and New Zealand.'

'We could hire a Winnebago,' he says, and we laugh, remembering a Frasier episode when Frasier, Niles, Marty and Daphne drove to Canada in a Winnebago and all did not, of course, go according to plan.

I walk through the dusk as we continue talking, and we both cry a bit. I'm a big crier. Ian isn't, but it's a natural release of the stress of the last three weeks.

Back at the house, when I've eaten, Jess messages to see if I want to talk.

'I'm here for you anytime,' she writes.

I message back and we chat for a while, catching up on news of Easter, when Daniel stayed with Jess and her family, at his English home from home. I'm grateful to have Jess and her family in our lives. She's like a sister to me, despite our differences. She and her husband treat Daniel like a son and are big supporters of his music and all his endeavours. Jess calls Dan the Accidental Buddhist.

'He's got such a Zen vibe,' she always tells me. 'He's so comfortable with himself.'

I tell Jess I still worry about Dan and am often frustrated by his reluctance to listen to parental advice or compromise on what he feels is right for him. I don't know much about the music business but I do think that if he wants to make it as a musician a little compromise might sometimes be in order. Daniel wants to make it in the music industry and yet is so unconcerned with his image and his looks. He wants the music to speak for itself and doesn't realise what an asset his looks could be if he played the image game just a little bit. But then again, his complete lack of vanity makes him who he is.

We chat about needing to accept our children for who they are, no matter how hard it may sometimes be. When the call ends, I try to wind down for the evening and let all my worrisome thoughts go. I drift off to sleep listening to Daniel's music on Spotify, holding my beautiful boy tight in my heart.

11 April 2021
Rain and food

And then came the rain. Cleansing rain, from the fringes of a cyclone hitting the coast further north. We're out of the danger zone down here. People have been told to stay inside, prepare for devastation. I pray they stay safe.

I do my morning exercise, read a little, then drive to meet Ian and Ben for lunch. We'll swap cars, Ian will stay with me for the rest of the week and Ben will go back to Perth. He has work and lectures and training all through the week. Life must go on.

Lunch is delicious. French crêpes, authentically Breton. We've been to this little gem of a crêperie before and chatted with the owners, a young couple who took a chance and left Brittany for the shores of Geographe Bay. They remember us, and we talk in French about this and that, asking them about the business and how they've adjusted to life Down Under.

'It's going well, so far,' they say. 'We're really happy. We have a much better quality of life than we could have in France.' Funny how they were drawn here, while I dream of getting back to France.

Classic French songs play through the speakers. I close my eyes and I could be in a little bistro on the Left Bank. Another French speaking couple come to pay their bill. The language fills me up, transports me to a different time and place.

Daniel lived in France for six months back in 2016. French was one of his majors at university and he spent a semester studying in Lyon. It was a defining time in his young life. He fell in love with Lyon, with French language and culture, with travel and wide horizons and new friends and possibilities. He fell in love with his future. It was in Lyon that the seeds of his musical dreams really began to grow. I think of Daniel now, of our shared love of all things French. I remember long lunches in the *bouchons* of Lyon discussing his hopes and dreams. I miss him so much and wonder when the four of us will be together again.

For now, though, I'm here with two of my three boys, I've eaten well, we've talked and laughed and it's enough. It's more than enough. It has to be. Ben heads back to Perth and Ian and I take the familiar road along the bay, back to our south-west sanctuary.

12 April 2021
Brothers and sisters

Ian wonders if I should tell my brother and sister about Alan and hits a nerve. When and how to tell them has been churning through my thoughts. I want to tell them, but I don't want to be pressured into doing it. There are so many people I haven't told, life-long friends included. I need to be in a place where I can deal with responses and questions and I'm not there yet. Ian understands my vulnerability, knows I only have the energy to confide in a few people.

I have no doubt that my brother and sister would send me nothing but support and love but I'm just not ready. We lost our eldest sister 11 years ago, and our parents not long after that. There has been so much loss. I don't want to be part of that loss. I think I only want to tell them when I know I'm going to be OK.

I talked this through with Daniel the other night because he's in England and it may come up in conversation with his aunt and uncle and I don't want him to feel uncomfortable. It's not that I want to keep it a secret, I tell him. He knows my relationship with them hasn't always been easy and completely understands. He's aware that past events have scarred us all, that the family dynamic is complicated and that I'm feeling the burden.

'If you aren't ready yet, Mum, save your energy,' he said. 'They'll understand when the time comes to tell them. Your comfort comes first. You don't have to do anything or tell anyone if you don't want to.'

He's a wise one, our Daniel.

I read somewhere recently that people who say family matters above all else are wrong. Those who matter most are those who love you and who you love back, unconditionally, whether they are family or friends. You need to stop thinking you owe something to people you happen to be related to, or people you think are your friends but who don't uplift you. You need to stop giving people a limitless number of chances to hurt you.

I don't want the sadness of losing my sister and parents to dominate my thoughts today. I need to let go of painful memories and disturbing thoughts. I have enough to contend with. I'm tired. I need peace and release.

Scrolling through the Chat 10 Looks 3 comments, looking for some kindred spirits, I find this:

I've had to let go of a few people who were causing me heartbreak … an aunt who got offended … a friend and her husband … too much, too hard. The one blessing of cancer has been the special people I choose to spend my limited energy with.

Later

I'm agitated, still. I need to stop torturing myself wondering who I should or shouldn't communicate with. There is no should or shouldn't. Will I never learn? Will I ever be at peace?

I escape with a classic film. *Lassie.* It must be a remake of the original, but it's not that recent. I recognise some of the actors. Peter O'Toole, one of the Richardsons, the Irish actor John Lynch. I remember watching *Lassie* films as a child. It's a heartwarming tale. An old-fashioned film that reminds me of curling up by the fire with hot chocolate on the winter Saturday afternoons of my youth. The comfort and cosiness are heightened by the rain that patters persistently on the roof, the fringe effect of the violent cyclone further north. It has destroyed hundreds of homes, we see on the news, but thankfully there haven't been any fatalities.

When Lassie has come home, Ian and I walk along the coastal path as day turns to night, sheltering under a tree when the rain intensifies briefly. It's cold and my fingers turn white. It feels like winter, not early autumn. I don't mind the cold, though, or the cloudy sky. I relish the rain and the wind, appreciate the changing weather. It's different to the monotonous grey that became too much for Ian when we were living in the North of England. The spirit sapping grey we left behind when we boarded a plane at the end of last century to start a whole new life. This grey won't last. The sun will soon be back.

I'm too tired to do much when we get back. I don't know what I want to eat. I don't feel like cooking. I pick at this and that and have a couple of beers. I enjoy the almost instant effect and relax. I rarely drink these days, so it doesn't take much to alter my consciousness. I'd be such a cheap date. Last year, I drank almost no alcohol, paid more attention than I ever have to my diet, disciplined myself to exercise every day, and now I have cancer. So, what the hell, I'll have a couple of beers and enjoy them.

Ian heats up some soup and a pie. We start watching *Line of Duty* on Netflix. Now seems like a good time to embark on a six-season series. There will be plenty of binge-watching opportunities in the coming weeks, I'm sure. It's gripping, and we settle in for the evening as the wind and rain rage outside.

13 April 2021
The waiting game

And so the days go by, waiting for next week, waiting for treatment to start. And there's another thing to do when I get back to Perth, something I'm trying not to think about. The "hot spot" that the PET scan picked up still needs to be investigated. The receptionist from the ENT doctor's rooms has finally called and left a message. I call back. I'm booked in with Tony for next week. It will involve a local anaesthetic, I'm told, so that cameras can be put down my nose and throat. Another bodily probing. I may then have another biopsy, depending on what is revealed. Will it ever end? I'm not sure what to make of this one. Talk of more cameras and biopsies alarms me. I'm hoping it's just a precaution. Hope springs eternal.

I feel slightly better today, after a more solid night's sleep. Ian spent the morning cycling. I read and tried to relax and exercised and prepped for dinner and generally did what my mother called pottering. I love to potter. I never get bored.

I can't decide if time is going slowly or quickly. I don't know which I'd prefer. Do I hold on tight to this last week of normality before the PICC line is implanted in my arm, and the zapping of my backside begins, or do I wish the time away so the treatment can start? These are pointless questions. Time goes at the same pace. My perception of time will make no difference to anything.

Right now, I'm sitting on the beach, the magnificence of Geographe Bay laid out before me, a stunning tableau of light and shadow, of gentle autumn colours and rippling water. It's late afternoon and the sun is sinking slowly over my left shoulder. It has drizzled on and off all day, but now the sky is mostly clear. The wind has dropped. Low lying clouds hover above the horizon in soft streaks of dark and light grey and creamy white. Birds swoop. I hear the occasional plop of fish jumping. Children in bathers search for crabs around the rocks, oblivious to the chill in the air and water. Their parents stand on the beach, wrapped in fleeces and scarves. I love this bay.

There's a sailing boat far away. I wonder where it has been and where it's going. Can I jump on board? Could it take me away? Could I sail away from this reality to a different time where my life isn't ruled by appointments and clinics and the daily grind of getting through cancer?

I'll head back soon and we'll walk into town for a drink in a new bar. I tell myself to keep things as normal as possible. Fight through the worry and fatigue. Live a little. Accept the cards you've been dealt. Play with the hand you've got. This is what I keep telling myself as the chill turns to cold and dusk settles over the bay.

15 April 2021
Home again

Today we're packing up to leave, which always takes longer than we think. And I have my hair cut a lot shorter. I like it. I feel freer and lighter in my head, my body and my spirit. I should have done this months ago.

There's time for one last swim in the bay. The sea is calm once more after the stormy effects of the distant cyclone. I swim out to the shark net, pausing for a while on the way in to soak up all the beauty. I'm up to my neck in clear, cool, refreshing, salty, tangy life-affirming water as I survey the scene. 360 degrees of wonder. My senses tingle. I make my way back to the shore and read on the beach for a while. Then, on impulse, I run back to the water, leaping through the shallows to plunge back in and lose myself in this ocean of tranquility, where I can forget for a while and feel at one with the universe. A perfect moment in time.

We drive the three hours north listening to music and chatting to Daniel, stopping for a family visit on the way. All is as well as it can be. Ian's Dad has had a good day. He does this. Rallies to the point where he thinks he can do all the things he used to do, then collapses, and the cycle starts again.

The dog is beside herself with excitement when we arrive home. Ben is asleep. He's on the 5.30 am café shift again tomorrow. He's used to it and is always disciplined about sleep. Good habits learnt long before I learnt them. He's a reliable employee, respectful of his colleagues, good with customers, diligent and committed. He's not a time waster or an idle chatter. I'm immensely proud of him.

16 April 2021
Back to reality

8.35 am

After a week of achingly beautiful sunsets, shimmering light, soft autumn colours and expansive horizons, I'm back at the hospital, waiting in reception under the harsh fluorescent lighting. I'm going to have the PICC line inserted. I don't really know what that involves, although I know it's the channel through which the chemotherapy will enter my body, as nurse Sharon explained after my surgery. I didn't realise until now that I would be going to a bed in a ward first and then taken for the procedure.

I've deliberately kept away from Dr Google since my diagnosis. I don't want to read about horror stories or worst-case scenarios or be subjected to ill-informed advice or any of the miracle cures that are pedalled unscrupulously in cyberspace.

I check in with a very pleasant young man called Daniel (great name) and sit for five minutes before being whisked up to another waiting room on Level 4. A heavily pregnant lady stands up.

'Ready to meet your baby?' the receptionist asks.

'Two babies actually,' replies the lady.

How wonderful, I think. New life times two.

Two days ago, I was cycling along the coastal path to Busselton with Ian. We pedalled through tunnels of green and salty scrub, the turquoise bay resplendent to our left. I managed the 52 kilometres there and back with relative ease. My body felt strong. I almost forgot about Alan.

Busselton has the longest jetty in the southern hemisphere, extending some two kilometres from the beach towards an underwater observatory. It's an impressive sight. We strolled around the revamped foreshore precinct for a while, past bars and a new brewery and restaurants packed with hungry holiday makers and children darting around the play area, squealing with delight. We spent an idyllic summer's day there back in January, blissfully unaware that a cancer called Alan was growing inside me, as the sun sizzled and the sand burned the souls of our feet.

On this autumn day, it was the perfect temperature for cycling. I used to prefer summer, but now I'm more in tune with softer seasons, gentler sunlight, cooling breezes and cleansing rain.

I'm brought back to the reality of my day room in the ward. I'm gowned and ID braceleted on wrist and ankle. Here we go yet again. The nurse completes my paperwork and talks about the procedure, which only needs a local anaesthetic. Dammit. No floating this time. When it's done, I'll come back here and have something to eat.

'Will there be tea and sandwiches?' I enquire.

'Yes, you can have as many as you like,' she replies. 'You can go home after that, unless you want to stay for the food,' she laughs.

Gosh this hospital is nice. If you have to be in a hospital, this is the place to be. I'm very lucky.

Soon, I'm wheeled into the theatre. I'm in Groundhog Day again. I shiver in the cold and am swathed in a now familiar warm blanket. I'm with total strangers, but I feel safe and cherished. The two nurses describe what will happen as they make their preparations, chatting to me reassuringly. One explains that the PICC is a long thin tube running through a vein and up my arm to connect to a larger vein that drains into my heart. My left arm is stretched out and my body positioned correctly for the ultrasound that will locate my vein. The other nurse explains that I'll experience a cold sensation on my upper arm while she cleans it thoroughly.

The doctor arrives and introduces herself.

'I'm a bit nervous,' I tell her.

She says all the right things and I relax as she gently talks me through what is happening.

'You'll feel a sting, as the anaesthetic goes in. It barely registers,' she says.

Then she tells me I'll feel her fingers push on my arm, which I do. I'm breathing slowly and deeply, feeling strangely calm. I have absolute faith.

'When will you start putting the line in,' I ask.

'It's in,' I'm told. 'It's all done.'

'Really?' I ask. 'I didn't feel a thing.'

When I come off the bed, they show me the PICC line on the ultrasound scan, running all the way up my arm and down into the centre of my body. Amazing. This is my lifeline, I think. They've given me a lifeline.

My upper arm is dressed, and I'm given a tube bandage to keep the outside of the PICC in place when I remove the dressing four hours later.

I walk out of theatre back to my ward bed. I'm signed off, then wheeled back to the ward and, as if by magic, hot tea and de-crusted sandwiches do indeed appear. I chat with the nurse about her training and thoughts about her job. She's young and competent, just the kind of nurse we need. Pay them more, government. (Pay teachers more too, please!) I marvel for a while at everything that goes on behind the scenes in hospitals so that I can come here today and have this procedure. So that patients every day have life-saving treatment.

We only hear the horror stories in the media. We read about what goes wrong. But every day, every hour, every minute, doctors and nurses and administration staff and porters and cleaners and caterers do everything right. So that we can be healed.

Ian picks me up outside the hospital and we drive home. It's just another Friday. I do some preparation for dinner, chat with Ben when he comes in from work, sort out some laundry. Then it's siesta time. I read a little, then sink into a delicious hour of sleep.

Later, we walk the dog and record some videos for Daniel's next release. DIY video clips. It's a stunning evening; the air is still, the birds chirp and caw their twilight chorus and the sky is aflame with another blazing sunset. On Monday I will start chemotherapy and the world is a beautiful place.

As I finish making dinner, I chat to Lorna in the UK. She's had the Astra Zeneca jab, her first one. Her husband had the Pfizer variety. Apparently, you get what you're given on the day, over there.

'The NHS is doing an incredible job with the vaccination programme,' she says.

It's the one thing the UK have done well, through all this madness.

We discuss the concerns about Astra Zeneca. She's not so sure she wants her daughter to have it, given the negative press. How can we tell what is fact and what is fake news, we wonder. Lorna was apprehensive herself, but glad to do her bit for the greater good. We yearn to see each other again, and to travel. We both miss travel so much.

'One day soon,' I tell her. 'One day very soon.'

17 April 2021
Acceptance

Autumn has retreated to the shadows. Summer dances back in, the heat of the sun beaming down from a flawless blue sky. I spend most of the morning reading and writing while Ben works and Ian cycles. It's just another suburban weekend in Western Australia. I feel remarkably OK.

Two Year 11 students have emailed with queries about the upcoming exam. One politely wonders if I would mind marking some answers. I'm officially on leave, unpaid leave. For 30 years I accumulated months and months of sick leave, never using my full allowance, and now I've just started a new job and have only a few days of paid leave available, which I used up following my diagnosis last term.

I'm impressed by my students' diligence and can't ignore their requests. I send back the corrected work and answer the queries and wish them well for the exams. I'm immensely fond of these boys. They won't know yet that they'll have a different teacher for a term. When I told them my news just before the Easter break, I explained that I wasn't certain what would happen. Maybe I should just leave it now. The school will sort everything out. I'm officially signed off. I have other business to attend to. But once a teacher … it's hard to let go.

I've been posting some photos on Instagram of our time down south. I'm a very amateur but enthusiastic photographer. I enjoy the creative process of choosing a scene, considering the light and composition, observing the colours. And of then selecting the best captures, cropping and editing a little, straightening up (I rarely use filters – the colours in Western Australia are vibrant enough). It makes me happy. I love colour and light and shade and texture and the glory of the natural world. I try to reflect all that in my photography.

I should really update my Instagram and Facebook profile photos now. But I'm vain, too vain. I look older, haggard, strained, thinner. My hair is shorter and darker, but streaked with grey. My neck is wrinkly. This is not the best time to be taking new photos of myself, perhaps. I'll wait a while and embrace my aging looks once Alan is gone. I'll embrace anything if I know Alan's invasion of my body will be short-lived.

I do my exercises, taking care not to weight bear on my left arm where the PICC line was inserted. I go to the shops, tidy up a little, potter. I've been decluttering since COVID struck and feel the urge to do more. I want clear spaces and clean lines. Maybe it's a control thing. I can't control what is going on in my body but I can control my home environment. I can throw out the old, take books, clothes and homewares to the charity bins. I want all the surplus gone. I can create space. Clear space in which to heal.

Late in the afternoon I walk across to the hockey club. The first person I bump into is our friend Alan, which makes me laugh inside, and then I feel guilty that my affliction shares his name. I think he'd see the funny side if he knew. He may find out one day, if I go public with this journal. Alan knows what I'm facing – it was his wife who whisked me off for a pizza last week – and gives me a hug and a kiss on the cheek.

Ben plays well and they win the match. Afterwards I walk in the dark for an hour, listening to the latest Chat 10 Looks 3 podcast and the beginning of this week's *Unlocking Us* with Brené Brown. There are words of wisdom here: embrace imperfection, accept yourself as you are, worry less about what other people think, do the thing that makes your heart sing. It's nothing new but the reminder is timely.

Later, in bed, I continue listening, but fall asleep before the end, soothed by the insights and gentle philosophising.

18 April 2021
Let the healing begin

It's just another Sunday in our leafy suburb. Lawns are mowed, cars washed, home maintenance attended to. I finish the book I was reading on my Kindle, prepare some food for the week, listen to music, stretch and exercise, chat to Georgia.

In the late afternoon we head to the beach to watch the sunset, our favourite end of day ritual. It's magnificent. It's always magnificent. I climb to the top of the dunes and survey the scene. Then a walk along the beach, home for dinner and early to bed. Tomorrow is chemotherapy day. Let the healing begin.

SUE TREDGET

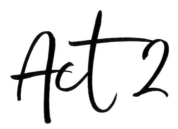

19 April 2021
On my way

I'm waiting to see the oncologist and start treatment. Chemotherapy first and radiotherapy in a few hours. It's finally happening.

I've been thinking a lot about people. People in general and some in particular. I find it interesting that complete strangers and people I don't know very well have been an enormous comfort, immensely kind. Passing acquaintances, my neighbour, cyberspace friends. Are my expectations of the people I know better too high? Is that why I'm often disappointed when people's behaviour doesn't meet my expectations?

When someone told you, years ago, how much they loved you and how they would always be there for you, anytime, day or night, and then they're not there and you have no idea why, it hurts like no other pain. The pain of abandonment. Is it my fault for expecting too much? For being a trusting soul?

I'm reminded of a Simpsons' quote Daniel used to love: "Expect the worst and you'll never be disappointed." Homer may well be on to something. It became a family joke, a one-liner we'd pull out if one of us was apprehensive, worried or hopeful about something.

I don't want to expect the worst now. I want to expect the best. I need the best to happen.

Simon has been delayed. I understand, but become agitated. When eventually it's my turn I'm flustered, unsure of what to ask. His manner is kind and reassuring but I don't take much in. After the consultation, Simon's receptionist escorts me to the chemotherapy suite waiting area. I see all kinds of cancer patients, some with no hair, some skeletally thin. It's confronting.

I'm too agitated to sit down, so pace around until my name is called to fill in yet more paperwork. More forms. I understand the need for paperwork and forms, but sometimes it's tiresome to go through the same questions and answers time after time. I smile, though, and try to be patient as the receptionist does her job and ensures all boxes are ticked. Smile though your heart is aching. Apparently the old adage "fake it 'til you make it" is backed by science. I heard on an episode of the podcast *All in the Mind* that the simple act of forcing a smile makes you feel better, by stimulating the amygdala and releasing dopamine, serotonin and endorphins. So I nod and smile in the hope that my neurotransmitters will do their job and trick my brain into happiness.

I'm called from the waiting room, led through to the treatment area and seated in what looks like a business class airline seat. *Where are the snacks*, I want to ask. *Bring me your finest champagne and make it snappy.*

My nurse arrives, smiling and kind. She's from the north of England, so we have plenty to chat about. The process will take a while, but she'll stay with me throughout. I'm being treated with two chemotherapy drugs. A double whammy. The first is administered through a drip as I recline and try to relax in the seat. I lose track of time – a couple of hours pass, maybe more.

I put on my headphones to block out the noise of the ward and close my eyes.

I suddenly startle and come to, blinking against the blinding white hospital light. I must have dozed off. A different nurse appears and removes the empty drip, explaining that she will now give me the second drug, which comes as a liquid in a pump she attaches to the PICC line I had inserted last week. I'll carry the pump with me for the duration of the treatment, and the drug will slowly enter my body. As this happens, the pump will gradually deflate until it is totally drained. The pump is about the size of a baby's bottle – I can hold it in my hand and put it in my pocket or my bag as I walk around, just as Sharon told me on my first day in hospital. The PICC will stay in situ until all my treatment is complete. The pump will be changed over when empty and filled with a second dose. It's all quite surreal.

I leave the chemotherapy ward, pump in pocket, to get ready for the next step, radiotherapy. So much is happening in one day. *Please may the drugs do their job*, I pray to no-one in particular, to all the gods of all the religions in all the world. To the universe.

To prepare for radiotherapy, an hour before treatment I have to empty my bladder completely, and then drink the precise amount that was determined at my first appointment, based on the size of my bladder. There's a lot to get used to on this steep new learning curve. It was explained that my bladder needs to be full to protect my internal organs from being fried by the rays. If it's not filled to exactly the right capacity the treatment could be compromised, or my organs could be damaged. OK then. Fried organs don't sound like much fun, and as for compromising the treatment ... well, that doesn't bear thinking about.

Conveniently, the chemotherapy and radiotherapy centres are five minutes' walk from each other. With time on my hands, I check out the cancer support centre which offers complimentary (and complementary) therapies: massage, pilates, Reiki and the like. I book myself in for a hand and foot massage later this week and a body massage next week. Why not? A little pampering goes a long way in times like these.

The radiotherapy session takes a while as the machine detects that I haven't filled my bladder enough when I first lie down in the treatment room, even though it feels pretty damn full to me. I must drink more water and wait a while longer.

'There's no problem at all,' I'm reassured by the clinic staff, sensing my anxiety. 'This often happens, especially the first time.'

The staff are unwaveringly calm, efficient, friendly, compassionate and seem to hit just the right note. I guess that's why they do this job.

Half an hour passes. I walk around the clinic, trying to ignore the growing discomfort from the pressure in my bladder.

Thankfully, it's second time lucky. I'm placed in a precisely measured position and lie as still as I can while the machine above me clicks and whirrs. The pressure from my bladder grows and I'm desperate to pee. Just when I think I can bear it no longer, the whirring and clicking stops and I head straight to the bathroom for release and relief. Apart from the hiccup with bladder filling, and the discomfort of not being able to pee for an hour before treatment, it's been a smooth operation. I give thanks for my strong pelvic floor, for all that post-natal clenching and unclenching. I'll have to do this every day for the next two months, so I'd better get used to it.

As I drive home, I'm hit by a wave of fatigue so intense I can barely keep my eyes open. I collapse on the sofa, sleep for a couple of hours and do very little else, apart from a gentle walk through the dusk with the chemo pump in my backpack and a symphony of crickets ringing rhythmically in my ears. It's been a huge day, but I'm on my way back to health. Back to life.

20 April 2021
Crushed

I have an early radiotherapy session this morning. I'm conscientious about sufficiently filling my bladder now I know how important it is and am back home for breakfast with Ben in less than an hour. It's nice to spend time with him. We chat about this, that and nothing in particular. About the final unit of his degree, which he should soon complete, musings about the future, his café job.

I work for a couple of hours on an educational collaboration I'm involved with outside school. I enjoy having some impact and feeling I can still make a difference; it's rewarding to use my brain and expertise.

Before Alan came into my life, I was asked to be part of a national Beyond Blue campaign. I've been involved with Beyond Blue as a speaker since 2015 and am passionate about raising awareness around mental health. That passion has in no way diminished now I'm dealing with a physical condition. I'm glad to share my experience in the hope it will inspire others to reach out for help instead of remaining silent, as I did for too long.

This latest campaign is to raise funds for the helpline, which I know from personal experience is what it purports to be: a life-saving service. The campaign coordinator has sent me the outline. It looks good. They're going to interview me and share my story with their national sponsors. I'm pleased to be involved and help create something positive from my lived experience.

Now I'm living another confronting experience. I hope that something positive can come out of this one too.

5.00 pm

The long-awaited appointment with Tony, my ENT specialist, stops me in the very few tracks I've made this week as I get used to treatment.

Tony thinks the "hot spot" picked up when I had the PET scan may be another cancer. I'm blindsided, and struggle to process what he's telling me. He's very matter of fact, telling me there's nothing we can do yet. I have to complete my current treatment, wait three weeks, and then have a biopsy. So that will be at least nine weeks from now. Too far away. Too long to wait. I ask him questions, desperate for reassurance, but he can't give me any.

'Is there anything I can do,' I ask.

'No, there isn't I'm afraid,' he says, not unkindly, but I feel brutalised.

I leave the rooms and crumble. I call Ian, distraught. He's equally devastated. I don't want to live like this. People keep telling me to be strong. That I am strong.

Strong is the last thing I feel.

'We'll get through together,' Ian tells me.

'I'm broken,' I reply. 'This can't be my life. I don't want this life anymore.'

The sun is sinking when I leave the hospital. I take a longer route back to my car as the tears flow. I walk round a small lake in the middle of a park and try to compose myself for the drive home.

The house is empty. Ian has taken his sister out for dinner. She'll stay with us tonight before an early flight to Sydney tomorrow. Ben is at training. I make some tea and toast and lie on the sofa, watching whatever is on, taking nothing in. When everyone returns, I stay put. I don't want to talk about it. I just want to block it all out tonight.

When I finally stumble from sofa to bed, I squeeze my eyes tightly shut and pull the duvet over my head, like a child thinking no one can see them. *Make it go away, make it go away.*

21 April 2021
Keep on keeping on

I have an early hospital appointment this morning to swap the pump over. Still tearful and distressed after yesterday's news, I call Simon, my chemotherapy oncologist, to ask his advice. He told me I could call any time, night or day, with any concerns. I'm put through to his message bank, but he responds promptly. When I tell him what's happened he seems a little surprised, given that the "hot spot" was tiny on the scan. He'll call Tony, the ENT specialist, and get back to me.

I drive to the hospital and the empty pump is replaced with a full one. There's a bit of waiting around but I don't mind. What else is there to do? I head home for an hour or so before radiotherapy. Back and forward, back and forward. This is my life now.

I talk briefly to a French friend I haven't spoken to in a while. Hearing the language I love is a solace. She chooses her words carefully, speaks with insight, empathy and compassion, with genuine care for me.

'Call me day or night,' she says. 'And put yourself first. Do the things that make you happy, look for joy where you can find it, put all other considerations aside. This isn't about anyone else. It's about you.'

When we worked together a few years ago our connection was instant. Our rapport, professional, personal and intellectual, brought me immense joy. It's rare to find a colleague with whom you are completely in sync, with no agenda other than to pursue excellence, share knowledge, keep improving, work only in the interests of the students. She's highly accomplished, and the teaching world is lucky to have her.

My friend's words sustain me through the rest of the day. I must keep on keeping on. I have no choice.

22 April 2021
Rollercoaster

I dream of travels, of my youth, of happy days in Spain when I spent a glorious term at university in Granada. My dream takes me to the Alhambra where I'm walking among the cool fountains of the Generalife gardens. The delicious reverie is cut short when I wake with a cruel jolt to my new reality, to the PICC line tubing in my vein, the chemo pump I now sleep with and must carry everywhere I go. The contrast between dream and reality is brutal. Unable to stem the tears from bursting forth, I curl into a ball and sob into my pillow.

When I'm all cried out, I brush the tears away and stagger to the kitchen. Ian is up and preparing for the day. It's tough for him, coping with work while I'm in this state. I wish I could breeze through it all, but I can't. I'm not a breezer. I'm doing my best, but I can't fake it.

It's now five weeks since my diagnosis. Simon calls to update me. After our discussion yesterday he contacted Tony. So many doctors, so many specialists. They discussed the way forward with regard to the investigation of my "hot spot" and have decided it would be best to do the neck biopsy next week, instead of in nine weeks. It's good news, I suppose, but I wonder why this didn't seem like an option during the ENT consultation with Tony two days ago, when he told me we had to wait, that he didn't want to jeopardise the current treatment.

Simon reassures me that it shouldn't (I note the use of "shouldn't", rather than "won't" – nothing in medicine is ever certain) impact the chemotherapy and radiotherapy regime. I guess I need to believe that and try not worry. But I'm confused. I'm losing track of the days, of the timelines of everything, and I'm befuddled by the whole process. My anxiety soars.

Shortly afterwards, the ENT receptionist calls to schedule another consultation with Tony tomorrow, and tells me the biopsy has been booked in for next Tuesday morning. I'm on the worst kind of rollercoaster ride. Everything is almost unbearably hard. I just want to lie down and drift into oblivion. I feel so terribly sad about it all, sad for our beautiful boys, for myself, for Ian, at this stage in our lives when we were looking forward to new adventures together.

I gather myself and prepare for the morning's appointments. I've booked a Reiki session at the complementary cancer support service. I had a few Reiki treatments years ago, when I was recovering from depression. I wasn't convinced about the benefits back then, but I'll give anything a go in my current state. Maybe Reiki energy emits special cancer killing vibes.

The therapist has a beautifully serene manner and I warm to her immediately. We chat for a while and I want to keep talking. As previously, I find the Reiki itself very passive – I much prefer a firm massage – but it's nice to lie down and relax. The room is silent and still, apart from some soothing music and distant noises beyond the door. I feel the therapist's hands barely touching me as she moves down my body and sense a change in heat at certain points.

Afterwards, feeling a little calmer, I walk to the radiotherapy clinic for my daily dose, bladder duly primed, and my business for the day is done.

Ben is home when I get back and we chat while I have lunch. It's natural and easy and very lovely, this time with my son. I treasure it. I treasure him. There's talk of a girl he likes. I tell him some funny stories from my student days and school trips to France. He's an appreciative audience of one. We're both adults now, close friends as much as mother and son. You do the work for 18 years, lay the foundations, and you reap the benefits. I'm beyond grateful for my sons and proud of our parenting.

I hope I get to parent them both for many more years to come. I want to meet their children and be the best granny in the world. They would both make amazing fathers, but that's way in the future, if it happens at all. I want them both to create lives that will make them happy and be content with their own version of success. And I want to be there to share it all with them.

25 April 2021
Lockdown

As of midnight on Friday, we've been in lockdown again. Two people tested positive for COVID and the government acted quickly. The lockdown is unsettling. I'm desperate to see Daniel and we're hoping he can fly home sometime this year. He hasn't seen his ailing grandfather for four years and wants to come back for a while.

Families matter. It's terrible being torn apart. The mental health toll of separation is alarming. The Beyond Blue fundraising campaign I'm helping with was prompted by a 42 percent increase in demand for their telephone support service. That's huge. We underestimate the mental health cost of lockdowns and separations and closed borders at our peril.

26 April 2021
Smile though your heart is breaking

It's Ian's birthday, and a public holiday. I've done very little over the weekend but I'm exhausted, despite the respite from treatment and appointments. Today all I need to do is have my PICC line dressing changed, and then it's back to daily radiotherapy. A review with the oncologist tomorrow, too, and the CT neck scan on Wednesday.

The "hot spot" saga continues to cause additional stress I don't need. The day after my phone chat with Simon, and the booking of the neck biopsy for Tuesday – tomorrow – I had the consultation with Tony, the ENT specialist. I was in such a state of anxiety that Ian took the morning off and came with me for support.

Once again, there was a lot to process, including yet another about-turn. Tony explained that the time factor wasn't significant and that the biospsy was likely to cause considerable discomfort in my throat for a while afterwards. His advice was to still have the CT scan of my neck but to wait until the end of my current treatment to investigate further. He went through all the implications and patiently answered our questions, without giving any guarantees of outcomes, as per usual.

After a couple of days considering Tony's explanations and processing the news (as well as lots of over-thinking along the lines of: *if I have cancer at both ends of my body I'll end up not being able to shit or swallow and die a horrible death*), I decided to do as he suggested and have the non-invasive CT scan of my throat but delay further investigation, which would involve another general anaesthetic and a full surgical biopsy. It seemed like the sensible option – I had enough discomfort in my life for the time being.

I'm doing all I can to stop imagining the worst, to put whatever the "hot spot" may be mentally aside and focus on killing Alan. One step at a time.

We've done nothing much to celebrate Ian's birthday. I've been too tired. I feel bad, but he doesn't mind at all. We'll delay any celebrating until I feel stronger.

This evening, I start watching *Gavin and Stacey* from the beginning. I've never seen it all. It's cleverly written, and very funny, and I become aware of something strange happening to my face. I'm smiling. I can still smile in spite of it all.

28 April 2021
Grounded

What if this is actually a gift? I don't know where that thought came from. Maybe in the night, probably in my sleep. If not a gift, then an opportunity to rethink the way I want to live the rest of my life.

I'm up early for the CT scan of my neck and throat. Another needle to inject the contrast fluid, a few minutes in the scanner and I'm done.

Afterwards, I walk to Kings Park, the splendour of nature a welcome counterpoint to the clinical surroundings I've just left. The fresh morning air is peaceful and still. I tune in to the sounds, sights and aromas, uplifted by bird song, by the towering trees and expanses of freshly mown soft grass opening up to wilder pastures. Endless bushland surrounds me. It's so beautiful.

I've always loved Kings Park. We used to bring the boys here when they were little for walks and frolics and adventures. It's a magical place. We take it for granted, this expanse of nature in the heart of our city. I should come here more often.

I lie down on a fallen tree log for a while, staring through the canopy of trees to the sky, feeling the healing power of the earth. Then I stretch out on the grass and do some yoga poses. The air smells of eucalypt and the glorious, earthy scents of the bush. I inhale deeply.

I walk barefoot for a while, relishing the primal connection through the soles of my feet, willing the planet to come to my rescue, to heal my body and strengthen my mind. To help me through this.

A friend sent me a link to a documentary about grounding, or earthing (actually just walking in bare feet, although you can also buy special mats, which smacks of opportunism), and about how the invention of synthetic soled shoes and our obsession with shoes in general is one of the worst things to happen to humanity. That our disconnection from the ground, spending most of the day in synthetic shoes walking on concrete and other man-made surfaces, is the source of many of our ailments.

I'm not sure about the amazing claims made about the power of the earth to heal us through grounding. But I am sure that connection with nature can only be a good thing, and I've always loved being barefoot. As I child, especially in the summer, I took every opportunity not to wear shoes.

After my barefoot wanderings, I walk back through the city streets to my car, stopping at a supermarket on the way. It's been a pleasant morning, despite the reason for the early start.

I tire quickly once home and do very little for the rest of the day. I'm listening to my body, moving as much as I can, but not pushing myself when I'm flagging. My mouth is starting to hurt from the ulcers that are a side-effect of chemotherapy and eating dinner is uncomfortable. I settle in for more mood-enhancing television. A few episodes of *Gavin and Stacey* take my mind off the discomfort – I can still smile through the pain.

29 April 2021
Ward 35: gratitude and rage

It's been a tough week. I'm back in hospital so Simon can check my mouth ulcers, which have become almost unbearably painful. I called his rooms earlier but he's in clinic all day, so he booked me a room as this is the only way I could see him. I'm in the cancer section of the hospital for the first time, Ward 35, which is rather splendid I have to say. In different circumstances I would pay good money for accommodation like this. People must die in these rooms, I think. I don't want to die here, splendid as it is.

Ward 35 is also known as the Harry Perkins cancer ward. Makes me think of Harry Potter; I hope it can work some magic. Friends of ours, whose lives have all been touched by cancer, have been fundraising for the Harry Perkins Institute of Medical Research for several years. We've supported them through the social events they organise each year and now I'm quite possibly a beneficiary of that fundraising. The world turns in mysterious ways.

After radiotherapy this morning there was a man smoking in the carpark, right beside a no-smoking sign. Against my better judgement I asked whether he had seen the sign. His response outraged me. He knew the sign was there but wasn't going to stop. Something snapped within me. Not only was he unapologetic, but also rude, selfish and ignorant and I told him so. Did he not realise this was a cancer facility for god's sake? My rage had no effect on the smoking man, who seemed, in fact, to find it amusing.

I walked away, trying to rationalise my anger as I made my way to the hospital, but failing miserably. I can still feel it. Why did I allow some inconsiderate idiot to get under my skin? It was his manner and the way he spoke to me, as much as the fact that he was blatantly smoking at the entrance to a cancer clinic with no regard for the patients. I'm annoyed with myself for letting him upset me so much. I need to focus my energy on repairing my own arsehole, not on some random smoking arsehole with no consideration for others.

Sitting in my hospital room now, legs curled under me in a comfortable armchair by the window, looking out at the gathering rain clouds, I breathe through my feelings. I'm waiting for Simon to arrive, hoping I can go home once I've seen him and avoid staying the night.

Nurses come and go, solicitous, bringing me tea and snacks I'm too sore to eat. One inspects my mouth thoroughly ahead of the doctor's visit, provides an array of mouthwashes and gels to soothe the irritation and advises me on oral care. I'd conscientiously read the information pamphlet prior to starting chemotherapy and have been assiduously rinsing with salt water twice a day.

'You're doing all the right things,' she says.

Another nurse arrives with an enormous care package of pillows and towels and toiletries and a luxurious mattress topper, donated to cancer patients by a mining mogul.

It's getting dark now and I'm hungry, but quite comfortable. I think of the depressing ward in a public hospital where my father took his last breath, of the hours my mother had to spend in stark waiting rooms before seeing her overworked NHS doctors and nurses and I feel lucky to have access to this level of comfort. #*blessedandgrateful.*

Eventually Simon arrives, just as I'm polishing off a surprisingly tasty hospital dinner. He's delighted with my restored appetite. We chat before he inspects my mouth and is reassured that I'm not about to collapse from malnutrition and dehydration. It's sore, it's not pleasant, but I can still drink and eat. He'll prescribe some strong painkillers, just in case I need them, and then I can go home.

6.23 pm
I'm still waiting for my medication to be sent up from the hospital pharmacy. A pastoral care person pops her head round my door to tell me all the nurses are tied up with an emergency in the room next to me. It may take a while before they are free to process my departure. She wants to know if what's happening next door is upsetting me. I hadn't really noticed.

'I'm fine thank you,' I tell her.

I hadn't heard anything untoward happening, but I wonder now if someone has just died in that room. When I'm leaving, I glance through the door and notice there is no longer a bed there. I imagine it being wheeled to the hospital mortuary and am less confronted by such thoughts than I might have expected.

Death is part of life. We can't live our lives fearing death, otherwise it's no life at all. These kinds of fleeting thoughts have been running through my head randomly of late. No one in my family ever really spoke of death. When my sister died it felt like the great unmentionable, her untimely passing. That which shall not be named. As my parents approached death, we didn't talk about what was happening. It was always uncomfortable. If death were discussed more maybe life would be celebrated more. Take the fear away. Talk about it. Name it.

The more I think these thoughts the more determined I am to live every day as best I can, to do this cancer thing my way.

I take advantage of the wait to lug my care package to my car. There's no way I can carry that and my bags at the same time. It's raining softly and the wind has picked up. The wet freshness feels cleansing on my skin and my already tousled hair blows untamed in the breeze. Light from the streetlamps bounces off the gleaming pavements. I love this change in the weather.

Back in the ward, I'm just getting into a Noel Gallagher (still a grumpy so and so) interview on *The Project* when a nurse appears with some painkilling medication, should I need it, and the discharge form. We run through everything and I'm free to go.

I come out of the rain and wind into a house filled with the smells of freshly home-baked bread and the evening meal Ian and Ben have just shared. They have been doing most of the shopping and cooking since the advent of Alan. We've always been a housework sharing family but they've stepped up big time. I'm not very hungry, thanks to the hospital meal, but I'll enjoy the leftovers tomorrow: fillet steak, gratin dauphinoise and a green salad. Delish.

30 April 2021
Finger on the pulse

What a day.

I wake feeling surprisingly good. My mouth is still sore but as the morning progresses the discomfort begins to diminish.

I have an early radiotherapy session, then walk towards Kings Park to commune with nature once more. The day begins to warm up as the sun rises in a clear sky. The smells of the earth, of life and growth and hope, seem accentuated by the night's rain. I'm enchanted. My spirits soar. I feel replenished, invigorated. My legs are strong. I take off my shoes and stride up the hill to the DNA tower. Then back down, stopping briefly at the log I found the other day to stretch out. This is my log now. It will become a spot to sit and ponder. Like my special place on the beach where I watch the sunset or the rocky promontory on Geographe Bay where I contemplate the glorious expanse of sea and sky.

On the way back to the car I browse in a bookshop and buy a novel. I have points on my membership card so it costs very little, which gives me a thrill. I've been reading a lot on my Kindle, but there's nothing like having a real book in your hands.

At home I have a work call to make about the curriculum project. It jars a little after the splendour of a morning spent in nature, but I do my best to quell my impatience. I need to make some amendments and review a document I thought we'd agreed on. It's no big deal, really. I'll do it on Monday, it won't take me long, but it's not where I want to expend my energy right now.

I work off my frustration by exercising. I want to keep my body strong. I listen to Daniel's music as I move, and it feels good.

There's a message on my phone from the ENT specialist. The CT scan results are in and there is nothing obvious to report, so our previous conversation stands. I call Ian to update him. He's thrilled with the fantastic news. I'm taken aback. It doesn't feel like fantastic news to me. It's just an update. The scan was inconclusive. I'll still need a biopsy down the track.

Shortly afterwards the ENT receptionist leaves me a message. After talking to the radiographer, Tony now wants to see me (I really like Tony but I wish he'd make his mind up). The rollercoaster whooshes down again. I should've held back from calling Ian. I want to stay even and calm in the face of updates, rather than perceive them as good, bad or fantastic. It doesn't come easily for me to take such things in my stride, but I'm making progress and Ian's overreaction has bugged me. I make an appointment for Monday, following my afternoon radiotherapy treatment.

Post exercise and shower, I'm relishing the quiet house and starting to prepare a late lunch when a freak accident shatters my peace. As I reach for a bottle of olive oil it slips and smashes on the bench top. It all happens so quickly. I look down and the little finger on my right hand is cut, badly cut. I collapse sobbing on the kitchen floor as the blood pours out.

Somehow, I gather myself and find a sterile gauze to wrap around the wound and hold the finger tightly with my other hand, wondering what to do. I don't want to go to hospital and have to wait for hours in emergency.

I call Henry, my GP, but he's not working today. The receptionist tells me to go to a private emergency clinic but I'm not keen. It's a way up the freeway and I don't feel able to drive while I'm bleeding profusely. I call Jacky from the hockey club, the nurse who lives around the corner. She's finishing up at the hospital and will come straight to me.

'Forty-five minutes max,' she says.

Relieved that help is on its way, I'm strangely calm. I don't mind blood. It's not too painful. I'm pissed off that my afternoon has been derailed, but I will cope. I do my best to clear the shattered glass and splattered oil while I wait for Nurse Jacky.

She arrives bang on time, dresses my finger to stem the bleeding, leaves to take her son to surf club, returns with sterile strips, removes the dressing (it's so tight we have to use scissors) and inspects the wound. Blood continues to flow. There's a big loose flap of skin and a deep jagged cut to the bone. We look at each other and I realise the worst. Stitches will be needed.

I refuse to go to emergency, I tell Jacky, but not in a belligerent way. She gets it. She's a cancer nurse and knows I need minimum exposure to germs and potential infections, all of which will be rife in a busy emergency department, while I'm going through treatment. We'll find a way, she reassures me as she rings around various medical contacts, to no avail. I try a doctor friend but she's at work.

Ian and Ben arrive home from their hockey coaching and umpiring. Ian isn't good with blood and accidents. He's good at lots of things, but not this.

'Don't ask,' I tell them both. 'Jacky's here, we're sorting it out.'

Finally, Jacky gets through to a medical practice close to home and I'm in. They have a GP who can stitch me up. It's only five minutes' walk but Jacky insists on driving and staying with me. It's great to have her company. We chat with the practice nurse and find out her partner worked at the same café as Ben for many years. Small world.

I nearly severed my little finger but I'm in surprisingly good spirits. Medical centres, clinics, hospitals, they are becoming my stomping ground, my comfort zone. The doctor, young and efficient, comes into the treatment room. She cleans and inspects my wound and the antiseptic sears through my body. Ouch. She checks for blood flow, strength and tendon damage. All seems good. The cut is in the middle of the inside of my little finger, just above the knuckle but I can push the tip of it against her hand.

'You feel strong,' she says, much to my relief.

The pain of the four shots of anaesthetic pumped into the base of my finger to numb it prior to stitching is indescribable. I wiggle my toes like crazy and tense my body as Jacky holds my arm to keep it still. Eventually, the numbing takes effect and the stitching can commence. Four are needed. I can't look.

'Great job,' Jacky keeps saying. 'What a great, neat job.'

I cling onto her, and she squeezes me tight. I can't quite believe my luck today, that Jacky was there, that she was free and able to come to my rescue, so willing to selflessly help me late on a Friday afternoon, after a busy day at work, at the start of the weekend.

It's dark when we emerge from the medical practice. Jacky drives me home. I can't thank her enough. Words seem inadequate.

'We must have a drink very soon,' she says.

Ian's a bit frazzled. I want to debrief about the finger, the stitching, the pain, the drama of it all, but he's not receptive. He's squeamish about these things. I feel a bit cheated. I managed to stay quite upbeat and I'm proud of myself. It's been a big day, the proverbial rollercoaster – scan results/not results, follow-up appointment not needed/needed.

I have cancer and nearly lost the top of my finger and Ian's pissed off at the attitude of the players in his hockey team during their match this afternoon. We're a bit out of sync and I feel deflated. I don't want to talk if we're going to argue. We don't often argue, but I'm disgruntled by his lack of interest and tell him so. We manage to de-escalate our exchange before it grows into something more than it needs to be.

I make dinner, the late lunch that was so rudely interrupted earlier. The steak is divine. I feel restored and spend the rest of the evening watching *Gavin and Stacey*, the first Christmas special and the start of series two.

I sleep soundly on my new deluxe pillow.

What a day indeed.

2 May 2021
Today's lesson

Happy May everyone. May all your dreams come true. May I be cured of cancer.

In the aftermath of the finger incident, yesterday was quiet. No appointments, no treatment, no freak accidents. An uneventful day, thank the Lord.

Why am I thanking the Lord? (And why not the Lady?) I don't go to church (my views on organised religion were formed by my upbringing in Northern Ireland at the height of the "Troubles") but I do have a very non-specific sense of powers greater than us, of being part of something bigger than we can ever comprehend. I have no time for evangelical style preaching, for narrow-minded so-called believers, whatever the religious label may be. Were I to invent a religion, I would probably mix the loving tenets of Christianity at its tolerant best with the spiritual essence of Buddhism, with its eight noble truths. Buddhianity or Christianism, I could call it.

I think of my mother, whose faith was uncomplicated. It must be comforting to have an unquestioning faith. She was one of those people who relish a rule book, who are scared to live without one. Me, I'm more the type to throw rule books away. I don't want to live by a set of someone else's beliefs. Sometimes it feels as though we are all living in captivity, dancing to someone else's tune, particularly in Western Australia right now.

Religion aside, God or no God, I will continue to send out silent prayers to the universe. Prayers for recovery and healing, not just for me but for our fragile planet and for man and womankind. For peoplekind. For people to be kind.

I know I'm not the only one to find people hard, not quite to the extent of Jean-Paul Sartre's "hell is other people". But tricky at times. Brené Brown, for example, researcher, behavioural expert and all-round over-achiever, regularly admits to finding people hard, so I'm in good company. She's also an introvert, just like me. It should be so simple. Use your energy, spend your precious time with the right people. Hold those you love, and who love you, tight in your heart, especially when you can't hold them in your arms. All my best people, they know who they are.

Then there are the tricky ones, the people who push all the wrong buttons. I'm not good at dealing with them. I've never worked it out. I'm a heart-on-sleeve, uber-sensitive, what-you-see-is-what-you-get kind of girl. I've never been good at pretending that things people do or say don't hurt or upset me. Even little things, like someone telling me I look tired, can be extremely unhelpful.

'What the fuck do you expect?' I want to reply. 'Of course I'm tired, I have cancer.'

But I never do. I smile and nod, despite the insensitive nature of the comments.

Why can't they just say, 'it's good to see you' or 'I've been thinking about you', instead of commenting on my appearance and stating the obvious?

And then there are the angels, angels like Nurse Jacky.

I wrestle, also, with the randomness of life. I've seen enough to know that shit happens without rhyme or reason. Everything is totally random. Good things happen to bad people. Bad people thrive and get away with appalling behaviour. Not all shit things that happen are opportunities to grow and learn. They're just shit.

I know also that if you think someone else has it all sorted out, that they don't have their own version of shit to deal with, chances are you're wrong. And as for karma? Well, that's a comforting myth we cite to reconcile ourselves to the wrongs inflicted upon us and others, to the tragedies that happen and the savagely random nature of the universe.

All we can do is our best in any given moment. And be kind. Here endeth the lesson. It is a Sunday after all.

3 May 2021
The power of words

Did I give people a bad rap, yesterday? To redress the balance, here are some things people have said and written in recent weeks; beautiful, kind, thoughtful words, words that fill me up and keep me hanging on:

You've got this and I've got you.

We're all thinking of you.

N'hésite pas à m'appeler si tu veux parler ou que je vienne te voir … Je serai toujours là pour toi, à n'importe quelle heure. Dès que tu as envie, contacte-moi.

Sending much love and positive thoughts your way. We are and always will be your Leeds family. Please keep us posted.

Sending lots of love and big fat positive vibes to you my beautiful friend.

You're a brilliant and strong woman and I love you so much.

Thanks so much for sharing your very personal information with me. You've been in training for peace and harmony and you have the inner strength and wisdom too.

Here if you ever need to rant.

I have plenty of time to catch up if you want some company.

Lots of positivity beamed directly at ya from me!

You'll get through this, Sue. Happy to be a support in any way I can.

Sending biggest hugs and love across the world.

I know it's not easy to do, but please shout out if you need help.

May God's healing grace shine on you.

While I can't know how you feel, I think I understand some of the space that you and your family are in.

We're thinking of you and send you our best wishes.

Your health is everything and we can cover your classes. I am glad you'll be focusing all your efforts on getting better.

And so much more …
And just to keep it real, some things that don't help:

I sent you a message and haven't heard back.

I know how you feel. My uncle/aunt/brother sister has just lost her/his battle with cancer …

What caused it?

Doctors aren't interested in anything except the treatment. They're not interested in nutrition.

Do you really need chemo? All those chemicals pumped through your body … all those toxins going into your system.

How will you know if it's working?

4 May 2021
Broken

A horrible, horrible day. Everything comes crashing down. I am agitated and anxious as I grind through my appointments, yet again. I'm in the worst kind of Groundhog Day.

First up, I head to the medical centre to have my finger checked only to find out it looks infected and antibiotics are prescribed. I just don't need this. While she redresses the wound, the nurse asks me if I got it wet. I tell her I did my best to keep it dry and find it hard to hold back the tears at this setback, however minor it may seem given the bigger picture of my life right now. It feels like the last straw on the camel's back. I am truly broken.

Back home I can't settle and cry on and off all morning. I manage to drag myself to radiotherapy, feeling wrung out and wretched. I see the nurse afterwards so she can update my records with the antibiotics. I tell her I feel rotten, and stay for a while. She's a skilled listener, I notice. So many people aren't. She gives me time and space to offload some of my angst and despair. It helps, a little. She tells me that all cancer patients hit a wall at some point, and this could be mine.

Next, I go back to the ENT doctor to discuss the scan. I'm not expecting good news. My nerves are shattered. I feel like I'm having a prolonged panic attack. He's running late, which increases my agitation. I find a quiet corner and listen to calming music while I wait.

Finally, Tony is free and gets straight to the point. There's mention of a lymph node in my neck. He says the words "as you know" but I didn't know anything about that. The words "lymph node" freak me out and I struggle to process what he says. I now need to have a needle biopsy on the node and he would like to do that this week. The results will take a week to come back. Then I'll see him again to review everything.

I'm beyond distressed as I try to keep my mind clear enough to mentally track back through this whole saga. My first scan detected a "hot spot" in my neck. I wasn't told about this in the first review of the scan with Charles, the colorectal surgeon. When I found out, the second time I saw him, he referred me to Tony, the ENT specialist, who told me the "hot spot" looked suspicious and would have to be investigated once the anal cancer treatment was complete, about nine weeks hence. Confused and distressed, I called Simon, my chemotherapy oncologist, hoping for clarification. Tony and Simon then had a discussion and decided I should have a CT scan and full biopsy of my neck straight away instead of waiting a couple of months. In my next appointment with Tony, things had changed again – I would have the CT scan but delay the surgical biopsy as originally advised.

And today, without delay, Tony wants me to have a needle biopsy in my neck, which is different to a full surgical biopsy, but sounds equally scary. It's yet another about-turn. I have no idea what is going on. Confusion reigns. Fear engulfs me. Despair triumphs.

I take the long route back to my car but barely notice my surroundings this time. I try to block out the stream of consciousness in my head. Is this it? Is 58 years my lot? I don't understand what's going on in my body; I don't know why it's failing me. I feel like I'm losing the will to live. I don't want to live if my life is going to be like this.

I lose it completely when I get home. I scream and shout and throw things around the kitchen and sob endlessly. I've done all I can to hold it together but I've had enough. I can't do this anymore. I can't bear the uncertainty, the layering of one traumatic thing after another, the seemingly endless about-turns.

People have been telling me how brave and strong I am, but I don't feel brave and strong.

I'm broken. I'm done.

8 May 2021
Tongue tied

I couldn't write this week. I've been filled with sadness and despair, going through the motions, attending at least two appointments every day. Yesterday I had four, ending with the checking of my finger wound for the third time this week. It's not healing as quickly as the doctor would like so I'll need to keep going back every couple of days, stay on antibiotics and keep the stitches in for at least another week.

I know that chemotherapy and radiotherapy affect the body's ability to fight infection. It seems ironic that treatments prescribed to heal the body actually weaken the immune system. There are signs in the hospitals and clinics advising cancer patients to minimise social contact, particularly in the time of COVID, to reduce the chances of picking up infections or viruses. For the first time I question what I'm doing. What if Jess was right? What would happen if I just rejected all treatment?

On Wednesday I saw a counsellor at the cancer support centre, but could barely speak. It physically hurt my mouth to talk about what was happening. The words were quite literally sticking in my throat; my tongue was well and truly tied. I'm not sure whether the session helped me or whether it just reinforced the awfulness of everything.

Themes emerged, such as my sense of being a burden and my ruminations on how to deal with other people, people whose attitude and advice I don't find helpful. I know I need to stop worrying about what others will think of me, about what they expect from me, about who I should and shouldn't tell about my condition.

There should be no "should", of course. This is my life. But I've been programmed from birth to worry about other people ahead of myself. I'm a Freudian field day. I wrote about all this as I emerged from depression, about feeling like an outsider, about the dysfunction and the deficit of emotional language within my family. I thought I'd made progress. I had, to a certain extent, but now that I'm sick all those insecurities and issues are creeping back in.

Both the counsellor and the clinic nurse told me to do this my way and put myself above all else. Above other people's expectations and opinions. The nurse used the word "cocoon". I like that. She urged me to cocoon myself and only interact with people who understand, accept, listen and uplift, with people who instinctively know all they need to do is be there, who know they can't fix me, who don't have some kind of saviour complex, who don't offer spurious advice, ill-formed opinions and unhelpful stories. With people who genuinely care for me, not those who somehow manage to make it all about them.

Like the French friend who emails regularly without expecting a response. Who has offered me her key and a room in her house if ever I crave a change of scene. Who, like me, often finds social interaction depleting. Who is there for me night or day. Whose kindness knows no bounds.

Or like the friend who called when I was on the beach earlier this week, searching for solace.

'I don't know if I can talk,' I said. 'I find it all so tiring, talking when I don't want to, answering questions I don't want to answer, questions that deplete me.'

She gets it. I can tell her this, and she won't be offended. Like me, she's an introvert and her social battery is easily drained at the best of times. We'll catch up for a walk when I feel up to it. There's no pressure or expectation. Just acceptance and compassion.

It's Saturday morning and Ian has gone for his first COVID vaccine. Astra Zeneca. The one making all the headlines because of concern about blood clots. Ian is unconcerned.

'The media doesn't report the thousands of people who've had no side-effects,' he says.

We only hear the bad news. Never the good. I'm bewildered by those who jump on every negative report to shore up their flawed logic about the evils of vaccination without looking at the bigger picture. I've never liked extremism and find the evangelical zeal of the anti-vax propaganda disconcerting. I'm pretty sure that a lack of vaccinations in some parts of the world has led to the reemergence of infectious diseases such as measles and whooping cough, diseases that were all but eradicated. No-one likes having a needle in their arm, but I don't understand the naysayers who show scant respect for the scientific research that has been saving and prolonging lives ever since Edward Jenner discovered that milkmaids who had contracted cowpox were immune to smallpox. I'm alarmed that disregard for expertise seems to be an increasing trend. We have social media algorithms to thank for that, leading the gullible down rabbit holes of misinformation purporting to be evidence or news.

The campaigners cite the erosion of personal freedom and choice. I'm no epidemiologist, but it seems clear that the vaccine is our passport back to some semblance of freedom. Ironically, the protesters don't seem to respect the freedom of those of us who choose to get vaccinated. Respect my right to have the vaccine and I'll respect your right not to. We need to live and let live (and vaccinations can help us do that).

There's now a vaccine, available to all teenagers, that has the potential to irradicate cancers like mine. Had it been invented in my adolescence chances are there would be no Alan.

As for freedom, well right now I'm a prisoner in Australia because of the pandemic. We need a successful vaccination programme so we can see our family and friends again.

I resolve to surrender to the new norm of my life. No amount of internal battling or anger or despair or fretting or screaming and shouting will make it go away. I walk outside to view the horizon, my horizon of hope, and am instantly uplifted. Some words come into my head:

I may feel sad, but I am not sadness

I may feel unwell, but I am not illness

I may suffer, but I am not suffering

I may feel angry, but I am not anger

I may feel despair, but I am not desperation

I may feel depressed, but I am not depression

I may feel anxious, but I am not anxiety

I feel therefore I am

I am human

I am here

12 May 2021
Reemergence

And so it continues. I'm in the middle of the fourth week of treatment and despair begins to lift as a few chinks of light appear in the wall I hit.

I had the neck biopsy last Friday. It was intense and frightening, lying helplessly as a complete stranger plunged a needle into my neck to numb the pain of the exploratory biopsy needles that followed, the ones that will determine my fate. I'll find that out this Friday. The doctor understood the fear I expressed as I lay down under stark lights in yet another sterile clinic. It was confronting to expose such a vulnerable part of my body. He could have been the Sweeney Todd of doctors, a serial killer in scrubs. A slip of the wrist and I could have been dead.

I've always had a vivid imagination.

I survived the ordeal. Thoughts of serial killers aside, I can't fault the medical attention I've received so far. I tell myself I've been lucky with that. Will I be lucky with the outcome?

My finger is gradually healing, but still needs to be checked every second day. Slow and steady wins the race. My life revolves around appointments, two or three on most days. The stitches will be removed from my finger on Friday, so I'll have one less appointment after that. Time is passing relatively quickly.

This week is better than last, when I temporarily lost the plot. Somehow my spirit pulled me through. I dug deep and found my way out of the pit into which I was rapidly descending. I withstood the storm of emotion, allowed it to rage and take its natural course. It was as if I tapped into some innate instinct that helped me let it be what it needed to be, and then reemerge rather than be submerged. Now, in the aftermath, a quotation comes to mind: "She stood in the storm and when the wind did not blow her way, she adjusted her sails."

People have asked me what I'm doing with my time, how I get through the days. I tell them I've plenty to do and am never bored. Occasionally, I'll forget what's happening in my body when I lose myself in reading or writing or sudoku solving, or cooking, or Netflix watching, or walking, or listening to music. I'll go into a blessed state of flow where there is no sickness or pain and I'm at one with the universe.

Last week, in between throwing things, screaming and shouting, I managed to finalise some details on the curriculum project, which pleased me greatly. Teaching is becoming a distant memory. I think of school sometimes and wonder how my students are going but I don't miss working. Probably because it's all I can do to organise myself and do what needs to be done medically each day and because I don't have the energy to control a classroom of hormonally charged adolescents. And I often get very tired in the afternoon, which is quite normal I was forewarned. Sometimes I allow myself the luxury of an afternoon nap, a delicious little European siesta, just as period six would be starting after lunch, so I wouldn't be much use in the classroom right now.

This morning I found out that the Beyond Blue campaign is being launched today. My story will be sent out to existing and potential donors with the goal of raising much-needed funds to keep the helpline open 24/7. I'm immensely proud of my contribution and hope the campaign will be a huge success.

I've been cooking quite a bit this week. I had a sudden craving for apple crumble with a thick topping and lots of cream, so I made one. Delicious. I baked my favourite lemon drizzle cake. Divine. And I made the best ragout ever. Dreamy. Paired with silky pasta, topped with a twist of black pepper, basil straight from the garden and freshly grated parmesan, it was an explosion of Italy for the tastebuds. Ian and Ben concurred.

'You should cook more often,' they told me.

Maybe I will. I love to cook. I enjoy the creativity of it. Now I have the luxury of more time to spend in the kitchen, even if I don't always have enough energy and motivation to create gourmet greatness. I must make the most of the times when culinary inspiration strikes. It's an act of love, cooking for your family. My boys are right. I must do it more often.

14 May 2021
A big day

Another big day stretches ahead when I drag myself out of bed. First up, radiation. I'm almost on autopilot now: Bladder preparation an hour beforehand (the holding on never gets any easier), a three-song drive to the clinic, a swipe of my appointment book to check in. The clinic generally runs like clockwork, and I rarely spend more than a few minutes in the well-appointed waiting area. Tea, coffee, biscuits and daytime television are provided to soften the reality of what goes on here. My name is called, I walk down the corridor to the treatment room, lie down, expose my naked body parts, close my eyes, listen to the machines whirring and clicking as music plays softly in the background. I usually count about three songs.

'All finished,' I'm told.

'Thank you very much,' I say. 'Have a lovely weekend and see you next week.'

I have a quick review with the nurses next.

'How are you going,' they ask me.

'Much better than last week,' I tell them.

We talk for 10 minutes or so and then I'm out of there, walking purposefully towards the next appointment, where I'll find out the results of the biopsy. It takes an hour or so, through leafy city streets and along the edge of Kings Park, then past an extensive hospital precinct to the medical centre. It's a blustery autumn Winnie-the-Pooh day. The kind of day I love. Perfect walking weather. I hear crisp fallen leaves crunch beneath my feet and feel the wind in my hair.

Tony is running late, again. *Quelle surprise*. I'm apprehensive but try to stay calm, listening to meditation music through my trusty headphones. I'm about to find out if I have another cancer.

After half an hour or so I'm shown into the doctor's room. He breezes in, greeting me warmly, asking how I'm going.

It's a huge anticlimax. The biopsy is inconclusive. I guess that's better than a definite malignancy. He feels my neck, then puts foul-tasting local anaesthetic up my nostrils and a camera down into my throat through my nose. I'm getting used to being poked and prodded and penetrated in multiple orifices. Camera exploration complete, he puts his fingers down the side of my tongue into my throat. I nearly retch but it's over before anything untoward happens. He talks for a while. All they have is a shadow on a scan, more inconclusive scans and now this inconclusive biopsy. He can feel something at the back of my tongue. It might just be an ulcer, he says, but he can't be sure it isn't cancer. Dammit.

He recommends "parking" all of this for a while, focusing on the current treatment and seeing him again towards the end of June. At which time, I'll most likely have another biopsy, under general anaesthetic, as originally planned, for further exploration of what the shadow on the scan means.

It's all so uncertain but something has shifted in my mind, and for some reason I'm not too perturbed. Alan was so clear. They took one look at Alan and knew straight away. This thing seems more nebulous, which I hope means that whatever it is hasn't developed too much and can be treated. Greg, my radiotherapy oncologist, told me he thinks it's probably nothing but agrees it needs to be explored. I see him every Tuesday and he's been very reassuring. Simon, the chemotherapy oncologist, also called me during the week to check in. Three guys called Tony, Greg and

Simon, four if you count Charles the surgeon, hold my life in their hands. I have the sense they really do care about me, these cancer specialists.

I leave the clinic and walk to a French café for lunch. The galette I order is disappointing, but it's nice to sit and read a real newspaper and feel like a normal person, not like a cancer patient still glowing from the morning's radiotherapy.

I take my time walking back to the car, enjoying the park for a while, walking barefoot amongst the towering trees to receive my daily grounding. I feel calm and centered as I head back through the streets to my car, stopping to buy a portion of soufra, a sweet treat to share with Ben later, and drink a green juice. I seem to have a Nigella-esque appreciation for food and flavours at the moment. I thought I might lose my sense of taste, but it hasn't been the case (apart from some unpleasant reaction in my mouth when I ate certain foods during and in the week after chemotherapy). I hope it stays this way. Food is such a basic pleasure, adding a welcome sensory joy to my days.

On the way home, I stop off for my finger check-up. All is well; it has healed nicely and the stitches can be removed. I wince at the sharp pain as the sutures are tugged out, and then I can go. It's been amazing, this assiduous attention to my finger, and so close to home. Despite the initial trauma, and the added inconvenience on top of cancer treatment, I feel lucky and grateful.

It's late afternoon when I get home. There's a delivery on the doorstep, a large envelope propped up on a huge bouquet of flowers. I'm intrigued. I put the flowers in water in the laundry temporarily, find a vase and open the envelope. It's a huge handmade card from a Spanish class I taught last year. I'm deeply moved. They have a different teacher now, but heard I was unwell and wanted to thank me for all I did for them and wish me a speedy recovery.

It takes a special group of teenagers to find the time to do something like this. They've drawn a picture of me addressing them as they sit attentively at their desks (not quite sure how accurate a portrayal that is!). They've written the main message in Spanish, with individual messages in English on the facing page. I sit with a cup of tea and read each message carefully, silent tears streaming down my cheeks.

This is why I do my job. These kids are why I continue to teach at a time when the demands of our profession make it increasingly difficult to focus on the purity of the interaction with our students. I'm humbled by their words. I clearly did something right with this class. I nurtured and listened and was endlessly patient with them. I mustn't be too bad a person, I think. Take heart, I tell myself, I've done some OK things in my life.

I transfer the bouquet to the vase and give them pride of place in the family room. The house is quiet until Ian and Ben return from their respective hockey duties. We all devour the soufra. Ian walks the dog. I relax as best I can.

Later, Ben has friends over for beers out the back, a time-honoured Aussie tradition on a Friday afternoon. Normality. They'll head out in a while, to bars and clubs, to a Friday night in the city. They chat and laugh and drink and play music. It makes me happy. Ben is in a good place. He's 21, with the world at his feet.

I head to bed listening to the sounds of youthful laughter. This is their time. Their lives are just beginning.

15 May 2021
The consolation of friendship

I've received emails from old friends, a couple we met when we taught at Barnard Castle School in the north-east of England.

We've only seen them a handful of times since we moved to Australia, but always pick up where we left off. It's a strong bond that will never be broken. Steve was a teaching colleague and his wife Marion is one of the warmest and most hospitable people I know. Barney, as it is affectionately known, was a close-knit community, a thriving market town. We worked hard and played as hard as time and age and work commitments allowed. We had dinner parties and drinks at the headmaster's residence and house feasts and all kinds of fun. They were happy days. Ian and I were newly married and building our careers in education. Daniel was born in Barney and Steve is his godfather. Steve and Marion also have two boys, who were teenagers when we worked together, and were an endless source of support and friendship in our early parenthood.

Their emails were prompted by a video Daniel has just posted. His music has brought them much joy, they tell me, through these troubled COVID years. Their eldest son lives in Japan now and they haven't seen him for two years. They think of us often.

I reply, telling them my confronting news, and am swept away in a tide of love and support when they each respond. Steve tells me he was so upset at my news he didn't know what to say initially.

'I wish you weren't on the other side of the world and that I could be there for you,' writes Marion. 'We are so far away but I am here for you.'

'… what a determined lady you are … come out the other end and write a book … you know how much we love you and Ian…' writes Steve.

I'm filled with love for these faraway friends. Hope of seeing them next year is one of the things sustaining me through all this madness.

As we wait to be reunited with loved ones on the other side of the world, we have to listen to a Prime Minister who can never give a straight answer to a simple question, who has the power to hold us all prisoner here for as long as he chooses, and a Premier who seems to be on some kind of ego trip and doesn't understand that you cannot "crush" a virus. You have to learn to live with it, and the way to do that is by mass vaccination.

16 May 2021
Control

I stay in bed for a while this morning, easing into the week ahead, reading, writing, doing a sudoku, watching TV. Chemotherapy will start again tomorrow.

I watch the news and feel perplexed by the human race. How can people in some parts of the world continue to fight, to pulverise cities and homes, to murder hundreds of innocent people, including babies and children, while as a species we are fighting the battle of our lives against the pandemic. Can people not just lay down the arms they've been wielding year after year, decade after decade, century after century? I will never understand.

Highly paid sportsmen get flown back to Australia, having taken luxurious sanctuary from the Indian pandemic in the Maldives, and will no doubt now be quarantined at someone else's expense.

Meanwhile, my son in London would struggle to find the money to fund an overpriced flight back to Perth, if he could even find a flight, or pay for the requisite two weeks in hotel quarantine. Not fair, not fair, not fair. He hasn't seen his grandparents since 2017. His grandfather had a stroke last year and is wheelchair dependent. His mother is going through cancer treatment. And he can't come back to his own country. It's all so deeply sad.

I've downloaded a book on my Kindle called *The Daily Stoic.* The essence of today's "lesson" tells us to control our perceptions, direct our actions properly and willingly accept what's outside our control. It sounds simple when you read it in black and white on a six by four-inch screen. Less simple in practice.

When so much is out of my control, willing acceptance is a concept worth working on. Hold that thought, I tell myself.

20 May 2021
One day at a time

My mind is on a hamster wheel, churning through the same old stuff, going nowhere fast. I wish I could stop worrying about things I can do nothing about and find a way to block negative thoughts from my psyche. Willing acceptance is tough. At times I'm filled with rage.

I thought I'd had my mid-life crisis when I almost imploded with grief and loss and plummeted into depression. I emerged stronger, more determined, less concerned and fearful. I found my voice and wrote books. I spoke up and gave talks so I could inspire others to seek help and never give up hope.

But here I am again, fighting for my life, in what is starting to feel like an existential test of some sort. I'm questioning the meaning of it all. My body isn't what I need it to be. I'm weary, sad, angry. I get on top of one thing only for something else to go wrong. My finger has all but healed now, there's very little sign of any scarring, but my right knee has now decided to balloon and stiffen. I think it's fluid. It hurts to move and I'm walking with a limp. I can't deal with the loss of movement; I need to walk every day to stay sane.

Sometimes remaining positive is so damn tiring. When I was first diagnosed, positive was the word that appeared most in messages of support. Messages I treasured. But sometimes it's just too hard. It becomes a burden, an unwanted duty you feel obliged to fulfil. Stay positive. As if that alone will cure your cancer. And as if a lack of it will be damaging to your health. That's a horrible thought – if I don't stay positive 24/7 I might not survive.

Just as I'm thinking some very dark thoughts, my phone bings. A message from an old friend from university days. She's a GP. I told her about Alan a while back and she has been checking in with me regularly.

'I just want to see how you're going,' she writes 'And send you oodles of love and hugs.'

The darkness fades a little and I reply.

'Doing OK, tired, chemo again this week,' I write.

She's on holiday in Cornwall and has posted some photos.

'So nice to see you having holiday fun,' I add.

We exchange more hugs and love. She tells me I'm remarkable.

'Really?' I write. 'I don't feel remarkable. You're the one who's remarkable.'

She's been there for Daniel on the other side of the world, calling him regularly when he contracted COVID back in March 2020 and couldn't access a doctor in London. I try to accept her compliment with grace – she's not someone to use empty words.

Our exchange lifts me up, even from a huge distance. Then Georgia calls. She's stressed about the move to her new flat, overwhelmed by the work that needs to be done. A kitchen and bathroom renovation, damp treatment, asbestos removal. She starts telling me all this a little tentatively, and then opens up more. She's embarrassed to have these problems, she confesses, given what I'm going through.

'Gosh,' I say. 'There's absolutely no need for you to be embarrassed.'

I wouldn't care if she told me she was upset about burnt toast, a broken fingernail, or anything at all. We all have our stuff. I don't buy into comparative suffering. One person's burnt toast is someone else's cancer. Just because I have cancer doesn't mean other people's burdens are any less real or significant.

I talk to Ian when he gets home. Tell him about my painful knee, my frustration, my darkest thoughts. He's always steady, unwaveringly calm and even. He doesn't panic when I tell him I'm losing the will to live, that it's all too hard. Even though it isn't easy listening, he instinctively understands that articulating difficult thoughts and feelings is part of the process. That it helps me to own them, to not feel ashamed, to eventually move through them.

He tells me he loves me. He's hurting too, I know. But he believes I will prevail. He has far more faith in me than I've ever had in myself, I realise. His love is pure and resolute. Sometimes I don't feel worthy of him, particularly when I can't mirror his conviction and equanimity. I'm full of what ifs.

'One day at a time,' he tells me. 'One day at a time.'

That's what I told myself when I fought off the black dog. I learnt to take baby steps, one day, one hour, one minute at a time. To realise that life is a gift. Not so very long ago, I contemplated ending mine. It's hard to write that, but it's true. I need to state it and own it without shame. I was in such mental anguish that I simply didn't want to live anymore. I loved life but couldn't carry on feeling the way I did. And I genuinely felt that everyone would be better off without me.

I couldn't see a time when I'd feel any better. I was tired of being trapped in my own head, tired of the racing thoughts, the painful memories, the grief, guilt, shame and inadequacy. I truly felt the best thing I could do was remove myself from the equation and rid everyone of the burden of having me in their lives.

I read somewhere, in the aftermath of Robin Williams' tragic death, that suicide doesn't end the existential angst. It just passes it on to the next generation. I know that now, but at the time I couldn't see straight.

If I survived all that, I can survive anything, I tell myself now and echo Ian's words in my mind. *One day at a time, Suze. One day at a time.*

21 May 2021
To hell in a hand cart

I drifted in and out of sleep all night, listening to podcasts and the radio, Ricky Gervais talking to Sam Harris about dreams, Brené Brown unlocking more parts of us, the measured tones of Radio Four.

I eventually surface and watch the end of the French news. I check my phone and see a post from a friend who moved from rural Essex to the even more rural Haute Garonne, south of Toulouse, several years ago. Not just in search of a year-in-Provence-style idyll, but of a whole new way of life. He laments the state of the planet, as is his wont.

'The world is going to hell in a hand cart,' he writes.

He's listening to Marvin Gaye singing about change coming.

'Marvin's predictions may have been delusional but at least we have music, at least we can dance and sing,' my friend continues.

I tend to agree with my ex-pat friend. The news broadcasts confronting images of desperate people swimming from Morocco to the Spanish enclave of Ceuta. Not just adults, but children, babies. An infant is rescued in the middle of the ocean. A 16-year-old makes it to shore only to be arrested by Spanish police and carted off to god knows where. In the Middle East, Israelis and Palestinians blow each other to smithereens in a hopeless, centuries-old feud that continues to decimate a beautiful region of the world, wreaking unspeakable trauma time and time again. Northern Ireland is rumbling worryingly towards a new incarnation of the unique history-never-teaches-us-anything conflict I know so well.

A more heartening segment of the news bulletin features the re-opening of French museums, cinemas and theatres, albeit with restrictions, giving long-awaited access to art once more. I'm struck by the comments from members of the public who are interviewed about this. A child, younger than 10, speaks of what it means to him to visit a museum again, after waiting so long. Others speak of the importance of cultural pursuits, of how it elevates our souls, and nourishes our spirits to be in the presence of beauty, of the importance of creative expression, of the awe we feel when witnessing the majesty of great art.

With those uplifting thoughts in my head, I drive to my morning appointments. All part of my new normal. Back home, I watch a documentary about Pink. It's moving and engaging. She's a powerhouse of determination to live her best life, juggling marriage and motherhood with an insatiable drive to create and perform. The clips of her concerts are sensational, particularly when she flies fearlessly, high above Wembley Stadium on her trapeze, not a beat or a note missed. I've never been a huge fan, but am taken aback by the strength of her live voice. If she tours Australia again, I'll try to get tickets, I tell myself.

The boys come home, a friend of Ben stops by, they walk the dog. Just a normal Friday afternoon. My second round of chemotherapy is nearly finished. The pump and PICC line will be gone tomorrow. Bring it on.

22 May 2021
Read and dream

The pump and PICC removal go smoothly. With my arm unencumbered – which initially feels strange – I head home with the weekend paper and curl up on the sofa as clouds roll in across the ocean and the rain descends. I've always been transported by the sound of rain and keep the sliding doors open to fully absorb the music of the downpour. May it heal and replenish me, I silently pray. *May it wash away my sickness and make me whole.*

There are some interesting articles: the latest on COVID, of course; fortress Australia; the scandal behind that Diana interview with Martin Bashir back in 1995; the increasing British royal disconnect following that Oprah interview and Harry's new career as a tell-all interviewee and podcaster; several enticing travel features in the magazine. My forcibly dormant wanderlust is reignited. So many undiscovered places, so many more stories to tell. I'm beckoned to Two People's Bay near Denmark, WA; to the Overland walk from Cradle Mountain to Lake St Clair in Tasmania; to the bountiful Barossa Valley.

As I dream of exploration, the rain continues to fall and the day edges slowly towards evening,

23 May 2021
Out of my head

Another rainy day. I'm sluggish on waking and stay in bed for most of the morning, unable to find the motivation to do very much at all. I read a little, then search in vain for a new book on my Kindle. Nothing appeals. I want something light but not total fluff and nonsense, something insightful and well written with engaging characters I can relate to. Add to that an intriguing plot with a few twists and turns that keep me guessing but nothing too graphic or gory. I download sample after sample but nothing grabs me. I give up in favour of sudoku and the crossword from the weekend paper, cracking them all in record time. At least my brain is still working well.

In the afternoon I transfer to the sofa and watch a series called *Collateral* on Netflix. I love Carey Mulligan, who plays the lead, and the rest of the cast is strong too. It takes me out of my head for a while.

Later I chat to Lorna and Georgia. Lorna has sent me a book so that we can read it together and have a two-person book club across the world. How thoughtful. We chat about our kids and her recent trips to Yorkshire and Exmoor, exchange thoughts about work and retirement and how long we'll continue in our current jobs. Mine, of course, is up in the air, given the circumstances. I hope my school will allow me to return on a part-time basis rather than go back to a full teaching load. Lorna thinks the business she works for may wind down soon and wonders what she'll do after that.

'Travel the world with me,' I say, and we laugh.

I'm more serious than she thinks. She asks how I am, of course, but doesn't probe and understands that I don't want to dwell on details.

Georgia is still overwhelmed about her move. She'll be starting a new job soon, too. It's an anxious time. We discuss books and she recommends a few. I tell her I've been finding some interactions difficult, and we mull that over for a while, wondering why certain people don't get it and others completely do. We sign off until next time and I look out the window into the fading dusky light. I walk outside and breathe deeply, inhaling the scent of winter approaching as the streetlights flicker on and the rain-soaked road glistens under the sodium glow.

25 May 2021
The circle of life

Five more radiotherapy sessions to go and then I'm done. I see Greg, the oncologist, after today's treatment and we chat about the end being in sight (as opposed to my rear end, which I prefer to keep out of sight) and how I'm going. I tell him I've had some diarrhoea – that's the chemotherapy, according to Greg – and that the area being treated is starting to feel very tender. I haven't looked, but it feels red and hot, which is only to be expected as it has, quite literally, been burnt every day for the last six weeks. Greg assures me it's totally normal and warns that I should expect the pain to get worse over the next two or three weeks as it takes a while for everything to settle, even once treatment has finished. When I tell him I was planning to head south for a while he wants to be certain I'll be fit to travel, and not in too much discomfort, so we'll review everything next week and I'll play my planned escape by ear.

He does a quick check of my backside and pronounces it not as bad as he'd expect at this stage. I'm tolerating the treatment well, apparently. I can't tell, because I've got nothing to compare it with. He tells me again that it may get worse before it gets better. Gets better. *It's all going to get better*, I tell myself silently.

Ben and I chat when I'm home and play cards and Chinese chequers. I win them all. He's not happy and I commiserate.

'You raised me to be very competitive,' he jokes, as if it's my fault he's smarting from defeat.

We've always played family games, both cerebral and physical. The boys and I used to play tennis, badminton and table tennis when they were growing up. They got better and better, and bigger and bigger, until one day the tide turned and I never won another match. Ben and I also played squash until the courts were turned into a gym, much to our dismay.

Both Ian and I grew up in families with strong sporting traditions. Through school and university and early adulthood I was never happier than when wielding a racquet of some kind, or a hockey stick. I started playing hockey again when Ben was six months old and enjoyed a late resurgence in my very modest but hugely enjoyable sporting career. I've long since laid down my stick and racquets to become a hockey and cricket mum, which has given me enormous pleasure over the years. I've passed on the baton and a few sporting genes perhaps. The circle of life continues.

27 May 2021
Life in slow motion

Looks like Melbourne is going into another short lockdown. More COVID cases are emerging. I message Marita to see how she's doing and wonder if I might visit her in August.

'You can come anytime you want Suze, for as long as you want,' she tells me.

I wish more people would get vaccinated. The continuing resistance and hesitance, on top of bureaucratic inefficiency, is making the rollout painfully slow. There are no effective campaigns, as in the UK and US, where amends are now being made for poor decisions last year regarding restrictions and lockdowns. It's been the opposite here. The powers that be are quick to introduce restrictions, social distancing and lockdowns but much less effective when it comes to administering the very thing that could render such measures less necessary and allow us to start to live with this virus.

An SBS documentary the other night highlighted how fear and suspicion continue to spread online. Trust the science, people. Vaccination may not be a miracle cure and yes, there are some low risks, as with everything, but it's the key to our freedom. Or something resembling freedom. Something better than being held hostage by this virus for the rest of our lives.

I'm sore now. Sore and very tired, with three more doses of radiation still to go. My backside is red raw. I'm not looking forward to the predicted increase in pain once the treatment has ended. It's draining. I'm depleted of energy and lack the motivation to do anything much. Once again I tell myself to go with the flow, but the flow is so slow and sluggish. The river is running dry and I'm wallowing around in the mud going nowhere. Everything is such an effort. Getting out of bed, preparing to go to the clinic, everything takes so long. I'm living life in slow motion.

28 May 2021
Let it go

I tossed and turned for hours last night, ruminating again on the slow rate of vaccination in Australia while other countries are moving towards greater freedom with Vax Passports in the UK and the Pass Sanitaire in France. I need to let it go and focus on healing and recovery, rather than worry about things beyond my control, but it's easier said than done.

My concern is heightened by the fact that my life is currently in the hands of the medical profession and I'm benefitting from years of scientific research into the most effective way to treat my cancer. It's unlikely that I'd have been born, had the average human lifespan not been prolonged by scientific and medical discoveries. I'm baffled by the vehement and unfounded scaremongering, anxious about the effects of continuing protests in the streets, saddened by reports of families torn apart by sickness and death and enforced separation. Will it ever end?

11.00 am

As I head to my penultimate radiation session, I realise I'll miss the staff who've been administering my treatment. When you see people every day for two months you can't help but form a bond. They don't just go through the motions of their work, robotically pushing the buttons that operate the radiotherapy machines. I know they really care.

When I told them about Daniel, his life in London and the pain of separation, they asked where they could find his songs. As I lay down to start treatment earlier this week, I heard his latest release blasting out of the clinic sound system, the volume turned up louder than usual. I sobbed silently as his voice soared above the whirring and clicking of the machines.

'We'll play his music for all our patients,' they told me afterwards. 'It hits just the right note and we need a change.'

How thoughtful. How kind.

As I lie down today, there he is again, singing the first song he wrote when he was 16, and then some of his more recent releases. It's both comforting and heartwrenching.

I'm starting to feel a bit better as the effects of last week's chemotherapy wear off. Constant nausea and frequent diarrhoea, on top of a tender and painful backside, have not been fun.

I've done very little this week and spent a lot of time horizontal, which is more comfortable than sitting. But today I have more energy and enjoy an afternoon of cooking and reading and piano playing. I'm very rusty but am still able to work through a book of sonatinas I used to play in my school days, at the height of my limited piano playing powers. Cooking and music. Creative pursuits. So good for the soul.

I have the house to myself for most of the day, as I often do on a Friday when Ian and Ben spend the afternoon coaching hockey. They'll both be out tonight, too. I enjoy the silence and the chance to just be, to dream a little, to read and reflect. I've never had a problem spending time alone. As an introvert, it is often my preferred state.

There's a storm in the distance. Thunder rumbles threateningly. I gaze out the window in awe as a majestic fork of lightning splits the heavens over the ocean to the west. I turn out the lights and enjoy the sky show for a while, as the rain drums steadily on the roof, splashes off the courtyard tiles, fills the gutters and pours from the drains. Blessed, sacred, life-giving rain.

29 May 2021
Quelle coincidence!

Another restless night. I kept waking regularly before falling into what must have been a very deep slumber in the wee small hours. It feels like 7.00 am when I finally surface with a start, but my phone tells me it's 12.34 pm. I must have needed a long, restorative sleep. I can't quite process the time of my waking and feel disorientated as I ease into the day.

It's Georgia's birthday. She's finally moved into her flat. I send celebratory greetings on both counts and she replies straight back. I'm still amazed that she now lives a stone's throw away from Daniel in a city of over 10 million people. She first met him in my swollen belly, about a month before he was born, and then again a year later when he'd started taking his first tentative steps. The next time they met, Daniel was two and we'd moved to Australia – her sister had also just emigrated here. Then there was a long gap until she came with me to watch him perform in Islington, the last time I was in London, in the days when we took our freedom for granted.

I tell her he'll be busking today at a market in their area. She'll try to check him out.

I spend most of the afternoon reading. Ian brings me the paper and I have a new book now, too. I'm enjoying it so much that I don't want it to end. I'm trying to savour every word and make it last, but it's difficult not to devour it in a couple of sittings. It's called *The Thursday Murder Club*, described in one of many reviews as "a remarkably accomplished debut … a genuinely funny comic mystery that succeeds completely as a crime novel". So far it's living up to the hype; it's a delight to read popular fiction that's intelligent and well written.

Ben has an early evening hockey match, an away fixture this time. I suddenly feel like going to watch him, even though it's been raining on and off all day. I have more energy than usual at this time of day, due, no doubt, to the length of my sleep last night. Ian is ploughing through a backlog of marking and isn't keen to go, but he's happy to drop me off at the ground. I see two friends when I arrive. We hug and talk. They are eager to know how I am. Today, I'm happy to chat about it all and give them an update. It feels good to be out and about. I've led a hermit-like existence for the last few weeks and for a moment I feel normal again.

My two friends depart for a Saturday night out. Ben's game starts and I find a seat on my own, rugged up with gloves, beanie and a blanket for extra warmth. The rain has stopped, apart from the odd speck of drizzle hovering in the beam of the floodlights. Behind me, another friend appears with her husband. I haven't seen her for ages. Our boys played hockey together at school and we've known the family for a long time. I used to tutor her eldest son many years ago and Ian coached her two eldest in tennis. They're called Daniel and Ben, just like our boys.

Anne doesn't know I've been unwell. She must have a sixth sense, asking gently how I am.

'You look good,' she says (lies?). 'But are you OK?'

I ask if she has heard anything – word can travel fast around our circles, but cancer isn't something people gossip about.

'I haven't,' she says.

I tell her I'm coming to the end of cancer treatment.

'I thought there might be something, you've lost so much weight,' she tells me. 'Although you don't look gaunt, your face doesn't have that hollow look,' she continues, as if to reassure me.

Sometimes it annoys me when people comment on my appearance, but I don't mind her speaking so frankly. She's everything I need her to be, concerned and caring and sorry for my ordeal but unfazed by the reality of it all. We chat comfortably throughout the match and afterwards she and her husband bring me home. She steps out of the car in the driveway and hugs me tightly. I've no idea when I'll see her again.

I talk to Ian about seeing Anne and fill him in on all their family news. As I prepare for bed I reflect on how and why it's so easy to talk to some people and so hard to bring myself to tell my family in the UK, my brother and sister, my own flesh and blood, about what I've been going through. As usual, it makes me sad but it's about time I freed myself from such ruminating. I want to shake myself, to slap my own face and snap out of it. This kind of churning never does me any good.

We're not the kind of siblings who confide in each other or share our day-to-day lives. I wish it were different, but it is what it is. I need to channel my inner Seneca and, like Elsa from *Frozen*, let it go once and for all. Come into my personal power, as the self-appointed social media gurus keep telling me, stop worrying about what others think, be kind to myself, unafraid to speak my truth. I'll tell my brother and sister one day soon ... when the time is right.

31 May 2021
Top of the tree

It's my last treatment day. I sleep late again and it's almost 10.00 am when I stir. I check my phone and am uplifted by messages from a few friends checking in. I still haven't done the whole mass sharing on Facebook thing, so not many people outside of my small immediate circle know of my condition. One-on-one contact is so much more meaningful. You find out who your friends are when you are sick – real friends, not cyber friends liking a post saying you have cancer. I can't go there right now. I've no desire to expose my plight to the world. Maybe I'll post a blog down the track, but not yet. I feel too vulnerable. Everything is still so uncertain. I need to protect myself for a while yet.

Yesterday was the proverbial sleepy Sunday. I dozed on and off in the afternoon, after a less replenishing sleep than the night before, read my book, did the crossword, failed to do the hard sudoku in the paper, watched some of those comforting Sunday TV programmes such as *Songs of Praise* (despite not being a church goer, I love traditional hymns and choral music). Ben studied for his final exam on Monday. Ian kept marking. Between TV and reading I managed to do some exercises. We ate dinner together for a change. I was hungry. Barbecued chicken, Ian's gratin dauphinoise, roasted carrots. Yum.

Now, I head to the clinic for my final treatment. Daniel's songs play through the speakers again as the machines click and whir for the last time. As I pull up my pants and hop off the bed, I can't quite believe it's all over.

There've been two staff, my favourite two, who've always taken an interest beyond run-of-the-mill small talk. Only one of them is here today.

'Thank you so much John, for everything,' I say, just about holding it together. 'I want to hug you,' I add, and we laugh and do the elbows thing instead.

In the waiting area there's a tree on the wall, the branches bearing messages from patients at the clinic. I'm told it's a tradition to write a message on a leaf on completion of treatment and place it on the tree. I write mine and look for a free spot. The branches are crammed full, bursting with messages of gratitude. John walks past as I'm scanning the ceiling high tree.

'Can I help?' he says. 'Let me help you.'

He's a lot taller than me and there's a space on a high branch I can't reach.

'Shall we put you at the top of the tree?' he asks.

'Yes please,' I reply.

'There you go,' he says, 'there you are, right at the top.'

There's more ahead, I know, but for now I'm done, my treatment is complete. I'll still have appointments but there'll be no more daily filling my bladder with a carefully measured amount of water, no more discomfort from holding it for an hour each day. It's time for my radiated backside to heal. Time to rest and recover. Time to just be for a while.

Ben is home when I return but soon heads off for his exam. I relish the quiet house, make lunch, listen to music, tidy up. Domestic bliss. Later I exercise and go for a short walk. I'm hoping to get back to longer walks again by the end of this week. I haven't had the strength or energy for the last couple of weeks.

Sarah and I exchange messages and then emails with more news and TV programmes we've watched. She loves *Line of Duty*. Ian is also a huge fan. He's on series five now. After starting series one I found it all a bit intense. I could appreciate how good it was, but it was too bleak, too depressing and confronting. The state of the world is bad enough. Corruption, betrayal, fraud and bullying are all too real. Maybe I'll revisit it when I'm feeling better. For now, I need a lighter and more uplifting form of entertainment.

Ian and I chat to Daniel after dinner. He got back to busking at a local market on Saturday and went to Brighton on Sunday with a group of friends.

'The weather was great and it was nice to do something normal,' he tells us.

He even swam in the icy cold sea. He tells us he's taking a break from social media. He's been trying to do the whole Instagram, Facebook, stories and reels thing but finds it increasingly soul destroying. Like mother, like son. He's been anxious about having to produce "content" when all he wants to do is compose and practise.

There's something very flawed in the notion that a creative person must also be a social media star, an influencer (manipulator), to succeed in their field. Daniel will focus on songwriting for the time being and, restrictions permitting, hopes to continue busking and get back to live performances sometime soon. He sounds in good spirits. Why force yourself to do something that goes completely against your nature?

I hate the pernicious nature of social media and the way it has become part of the fabric of our lives. The reducing of our experiences to 15-second video clips, carefully curated photos, cliched soundbites, annoying exhortations to do this, that and the other, and not to do the opposite. Three ways to achieve your goals. Five ways to fulfil your dreams. Seven ways to find true happiness. The ever-decreasing attention span of the young. If I see a beautiful sunset and don't post about it, did it really happen? We post, therefore we are.

I'm in no doubt about Daniel's talent but wonder if that's enough to break through in the music industry. I sometimes gently suggest he needs a Plan B, should his musical dreams fall short. He used to tell me there was no Plan B, but now he's a little more receptive. He tells me he'll know when he needs to explore other avenues for his creative talent. It doesn't seem right that someone with so much passion and ability can't find a way through. He's too nice a person, too deep a thinker, to find fulfillment in an online world.

As I'm getting ready for bed, Georgia calls to congratulate me on finishing treatment.

'Thanks, I'm glad that part's over but I'm not out of the woods yet,' I tell her, before shifting the focus away from me. I don't want to get into a long discussion and speculate about what lies ahead.

'And how are you?' I ask.

Georgia has two siblings, a brother and a sister, and often finds herself in tears over something they've said or not said, done or not done, an insensitive remark, an unkind word, that shows how little they understand her, that reinforces the disconnect between them. Today, she's upset that they haven't been helpful during the upheaval of her move and were dismissive of the anxiety it caused her. I'm happy to be a sounding board and let her talk it out of her system.

Everyone has their stuff. I think of my own brother and sister and suddenly want to reach out to them, to reconnect with my family in the UK, to make up for lost time, to see my nieces and nephews – and great nieces and nephews. I'm hoping for better times ahead, for open borders and joyful reunions. I remember that scene from *Billy Elliott* when the dancers are rehearsing to *The Sun Will Come Out Tomorrow*, and Julie Walters, cigarette in hand, quips, "fat chance". It always makes me smile in a bittersweet way. I hope there's more than a fat chance.

As I drift off to sleep I think of my boy on the other side of the world, of family and friends near and far, and hold them all close in my heart.

Intermission

1 June 2021
Winter

It's officially winter. Happy winter to all in the Southern Hemisphere. And happy summer to all on the other side of the globe. May the changing seasons bring us joy, love and light and help us make changes in our lives, if that is what we need.

I love winter in Perth. It never gets too bleak, but there is wind and rain a-plenty, to satisfy my wild Irish soul, and stormy days to stir the spirit. I also love those days when the searing blue sky contrasts with the almost icy morning and evening temperatures. People are rather loose with the term "freezing" here. They should try living in County Durham or Northern Ireland. Then they'd find out all about freezing. I can't ever remember the temperature getting as low as zero degrees here. Four degrees is a very cold night. Freezing is a relative term. Relative, here, to summer temperatures that sometimes nudge over 40. So, I just smile and nod when someone comments on the "freezing" weather.

That said, we do sometimes get snow further south, in the Stirling Ranges. And occasionally, very occasionally, I've seen a film of almost-white dew on the grass in the morning. Now and again, we get hail as big as golf balls. There's certainly plenty of weather in Perth. Lots of change and contrast. It's funny, the variety of perceptions people have. When we were planning to emigrate to Australia, a colleague in England told me she couldn't live in a place with no change in the seasons.

Each season here announces itself quite clearly. As Gerard Manley Hopkins wrote, "nothing is so beautiful as spring" in Western Australia. We have some of the rarest, most diverse spring flower displays on the planet, and while our autumn colours may not quite rival those of fall in New England, the mellow fruitfulness, the golds and yellows and russets and reds abound.

My thoughts hover around seasons and weather today, but I'm not feeling good. I'm sore and tired and once again can't bring myself to do much. So I don't. I rest and read and play the piano and watch TV. That's all I can face. I was planning a trip to IKEA for some home organisation therapy, but that will have to wait. I feel I may be falling into a hole again. Treatment is finished but there's a long way to go. And I'm worried about Daniel after our recent chats.

When does it end, this maternal concern? Probably never. We have another long talk today. He's been feeling anxious. I know all about anxiety and listen attentively. I'm reluctant to offer too much advice when he clearly needs to talk. I love this boy so much it tears me in two sometimes. I want to make everything right for him, but he needs to find his own way. I try to steer him towards taking more action with his songwriting, putting himself out there, knocking on doors, whether real or virtual.

I tell him I've been listening to a podcast called *We Write the Songs*. Gary Barlow interviews some of the world's most successful songwriters about their craft. It's fascinating. Daniel would learn a lot from it, but sometimes he appears reluctant to take on ideas or advice. Or maybe it's all just too daunting. Finding your way and knowing what to do with the bombardment of online advice must be completely overwhelming. I don't know anything about the music business, but I do know he can't do this alone. He needs to find his musical tribe, to connect with like minds. He needs to hustle, persist, network, make contacts and follow them up, then hustle some more.

I'm not sure if it's him, though, the hustle, if he has a thick enough skin to withstand rejection after rejection, to avoid taking criticism to heart. I'm worried, sad and frustrated on his behalf. It's hard to want to help so badly and know you really can't. He must do life his own way, and if that means he won't ever be the successful singer-songwriter he dreams of becoming, well then so be it. He'll still be one awesome human.

2 June 2021
Words and music

I feel a little stronger this morning. A package has arrived, the book Lorna told me she would send. We'll both read it, then discuss it, in our own special trans-global book club. It's called *This is Happiness*, by Niall Williams, an Irish author. She was listening to it on Audible and it made her smile and think of me.

I've always loved reading and storytelling. There's nothing quite like losing yourself in a good story well told. I still have some books from my childhood, books my mother used to read to me. As I was going through some old boxes in our shed during a COVID clearout, I came upon a collection of bedtime tales for the under sixes called *Tell me a Story*. I loved that book. If I close my eyes and concentrate hard, I can almost hear my mother's flat northern English vowels as she reads it softly to me while I curl up under the covers, drifting to another time and place, another world. It's a bit battered and torn now, but I'll treasure it forever.

As a child I used to make up stories and tell them to my collection of teddy bears, dolls and other stuffed animals. I had an elephant called Lorna I just loved. I smile at the memory, given my friend's name. I had a wild imagination, filled with evil witches and dragons and all kinds of magical creatures. My father would make up leprechaun stories for me. Tales of shoemaking and dancing around fairy rings and pots of gold and crafty tricks to fool humankind.

As soon as I could read on my own there was no stopping me. I always had my head in a book. Anne of Green Gables, such a delight. The *Narnia* books. *Tom's Midnight Garden*, *The Secret Garden* and other childhood classics. *The Famous Five* and all the Enid Blyton books based in schools, *Mallory Towers* and the like. Nail-biting games of lacrosse. Pillow fights and midnight feasts. French teachers with thick accents and hair in tight buns. Tales of adventure and discovery. Potholes and underground streams. Smugglers and robbers. Picnics with lashings of ginger beer. Bliss.

While that girl who read as if her life depended on it (it probably did) still burns within me, I need to fan those flames. That's one of the seasonal changes I want to make. I need to read and learn as much as I can and follow through on what I started when I published my own books in 2017. I let it slide. It seemed too hard to keep promoting myself through social media. Daniel and I are so alike in that respect. We both need to find a way to live our best creative lives, regardless of likes or followers or the beauty of our Insta grids. My concern for Daniel, my anxiety about his anxiety, is just a mirror of my own inertia and fear of pursuing my dreams.

What will my story be now, I wonder. How will it end?

I spend a couple of hours in the kitchen, arranging food and utensils in cupboards and drawers, reorganising spices. I want to have something to do, to feel useful. I can't control what is happening to my body, but I can bring a little domestic order to the home. I can control where the cumin, coriander and cinnamon are stored, at least until someone forgets to put them back where they came from. Then I can get annoyed and have a rant before taking control of the spices once more and feeling useful again.

As I potter, I listen to an R.E.M playlist I've just created, including many songs from the early 1980s, long before *Losing my Religion* hit the airwaves. The soaring melancholy of Michael Stipe's vocals mirrors my mood. It's soothing. I've always loved sad vocals, melodic keys, nostalgic lyrics. I used to listen to the Smiths when feeling lovelorn and abandoned in my student days, Morrissey's misery somehow affirming mine and making it more bearable. I'm not miserable now (heaven knows) but I'm in need of the solace that music never fails to provide.

3 June 2021
Tidy house, tidy mind

I get up promptly to sort out the house for the cleaners, tidying up so they can do their thing. We employed our cleaners, a husband-and-wife team, a couple of years ago. They come once a week, a luxury I know, but more than worth it. Now that my income is on hold, I wonder how much longer we can justify the expense, but Ian insists we keep them on. It's always nice to start the weekend with a clean and orderly house. It's a small but important pleasure that cannot be underestimated. Tidy house, tidy mind.

I head to the beach for a couple of hours while the cleaners do their thing. It's a blue-sky perfect winter's day. I enjoy the chill in the air as I sit and listen to another podcast about songwriting and plan to share and discuss it with Daniel. When the podcast ends, I walk along the coastal path as the waves break and crash in a timeless cycle, an eternal ebb and flow. Seagulls soar and swoop. Fitter and faster walkers overtake me with friendly nods. We're all here doing our thing, being in nature, moving our bodies, raising our heart rates.

I return to my sparkly clean house, drink tea, make a sandwich and prepare for a Zoom call with Fred, my website creator. We've been trying to set up this meeting for a while. It's good to see him. He talks me through the revamp of my site, shows me how to edit and change text under the new system. I'm a technophobe from way back but it doesn't seem too hard. He's endlessly patient. We discuss making more changes, altering titles, streamlining sections, focusing more on marketing, promotion and selling my books. In my dreams I'd make my living as a writer. Fred is there to help me. It's up to me to find the self-discipline and determination to make it happen, this writing life that I crave.

Ian and Ben arrive home. We have a long weekend. I spend time working on my website while Fred's instructions are fresh in my mind. I'm able to make some edits and resolve to work on it more regularly so that I don't forget how to do it. As with anything, practice makes perfect. I have the time now. I have no excuse.

Time flies when I'm focused and a couple of hours have passed when I stop working, editing and thinking about writing. Ben walks the dog, then heads out to watch footy at the pub with friends. Ian goes to the gym while I do some exercise before dinner. I'm eating regularly, but far less than I used to. I weigh myself every day, hoping, for the first time in my life, that the number displayed won't have dropped too much.

I'm reading a new book on my Kindle, *The Mistake* by Katie McMahon. It's her debut novel and comes highly recommended by Liane Moriarty. I met her once, Liane that is. She signed all my books – I have every one of hers – and she gave me some writing advice. I was totally starstruck. I have a photo of us together somewhere on my phone. I must dig it out and use it for inspiration. I'm really enjoying *The Mistake*. It's just the kind of book I would like to write I think, as the Kindle slips from my hands onto my pillow and I fall asleep.

4 June 2021
A good day

Ian and Ben leave early for a day visiting Ian's parents, and I wake to a quiet house. It's another WA perfect winter's day, chilly in the shade, warmer in the sun, blue sky forever, yellow, red and orange leaves dropping on the lawn, distant weekend noises drifting through the pure, clear air.

As I'm drinking my morning coffee, Marita messages.

'Do you want to chat?'

What perfect timing. We spend an hour or so updating each other. Today I'm happy to talk freely about how I'm doing. I don't always want to talk about it, but with Marita it's so easy. There's no pressure to share too much, or anything at all. We move through different topics, as is our wont – family, her work, the Melbourne lockdown, the news of the day. It's like the most comforting cup of tea with the most delicious biscuits. I feel replenished when we finish talking, ready to face the day.

I head to the beach in the early afternoon and have my first dip in the ocean since my diagnosis. It's blissful. I play around in the waves for a while, then swaddle myself in warm clothes and lie face down close to the dunes, relishing the winter sun on my back.

Later in the afternoon another friend calls. She and her husband have been forced to quarantine after a work trip to Melbourne. My plans to visit them next week, at their place down south, must be put on hold for now. No matter. We share our exasperation with the state of the world and the unpredictability of everything and conclude, as always, that all we can do at any given moment, through any given situation, is our best. We hang up, promising to speak again very soon. I take the dog out for a short walk in the twilight as another day draws to a close.

6 June 2021
Afternoon delight

It's six days since treatment ended. Something amazing happens. After a morning of reading, writing, exercise, a jump in the waves and an exquisite I've-almost-forgotten-I'm-fighting-cancer time on the beach, I realise I feel less tired than I have in a while. I don't quite know what to do with my extra energy. Then I have an idea.

I tell Ian I need his help with something. He thinks it means I want him to move some furniture (household reconfiguring is a hobby of mine) and reluctantly tears himself away from some scintillating YouTube lecture about particle physics. I actually mean I want to him to help me find out if my body can still do the things it used to do, pre-Alan, on a not-particularly-frequent-but-still-acceptably-regular-after-27-years-of-marriage basis. It takes a moment for the penny to drop.

I'm filled with fear. My body has changed. That whole area is very tender, still burnt and raw from the radiation. I worry that Ian won't find me attractive, may even be repelled, that it will hurt, that I won't be able to respond.

I needn't have worried.

'You're beautiful,' Ian tells me. 'You're always beautiful to me,' he says as he cradles my ravaged body.

I know they aren't just empty words. I know that my man loves me to the moon and back and always will. I often don't feel worthy of that love. Nor do I feel in any way beautiful, but eye of the beholder and all that. He doesn't want to hurt me or do anything to make me feel uncomfortable.

'Your body has been through a huge trauma,' he tells me.

But I want to try. I'm not overcome with lust, but I want to know. I want to feel something, to feel human. I'm tentative but able to respond a little. There are no thunderbolts, lightning doesn't quite strike, the earth does not move, but everything seems to be in good working order. It's a start, at least. And Ian, well Ian is over the moon. Bloody men. It's so easy for them. He's in fine working order and can't wipe the smile off his face for the rest of the day.

I make Thai fishcakes for dinner, a family favourite, and we watch *Spicks and Specks*, the latest series. I don't rise to the bait when Ian makes politically incorrect comments about the contestants and Adam Hills. We have a one degree of separation connection to Adam Hills; Daniel met him and his wife, Ally McGregor, when he first arrived in London. Ally took Daniel to a function at Australia House, Adam took him to see Russell Crowe's band and on another occasion they met up to watch Ally perform at the Edinburgh festival. Since Edinburgh, they've had one or two online exchanges but early suggestions that Adam would introduce him to some music industry people did not eventuate. He's a busy man, Adam, flying back and forward across the world, even in the time of COVID, so a struggling Aussie singer-songwriter is understandably not high on his agenda.

Ian and Ben clear the table, load the dishwasher and tidy up. We talk about the week ahead. I catch the end of *MasterChef* and watch some of the French Open tennis.

Take Alan out of the equation and it's been a pretty perfect Sunday.

7 June 2021
Find the joy

Despite the quasi-perfection of yesterday, I can't sleep. My mind is racing with ideas for books and blogs and all things creative. Do I or don't I start posting some of these diary entries I've been writing? Do I tell the world (on my public Facebook page, or all 167 of my Facebook friends) about my illness? Am I strong enough to be vulnerable? Will I regret oversharing? Will I find it all too overwhelming and exhausting?

It's hard not knowing how my story ends. I'm right in the middle of it. Is it too soon to put it out there when I don't know if I'll make it? I was comfortable sharing my diagnosis with the Chat 10 group right at the start, drew strength from the virtual support and found the courage to face what lay ahead. My cry for help was answered with the reassurance I sought: I was not alone. But I didn't have the energy or inclination to keep checking in. And I'm not yet sure if I'm ready to share Alan with the world.

I get up and wander around the house, my brain fizzing. I try to switch off by reading my current Kindle book and finish it with regret – I didn't want it to end, and I don't have another lined up. I hate that. I think I finally fall asleep around 5 am. Ian wakes me at 9.00 am to see if I want a coffee and makes some quip about a reprise of yesterday's activity.

'Don't push your luck,' I tell him. 'And yes, I need coffee big time so make it snappy.'

He laughs.

I stay in bed and he brings me a triple shot long black, courtesy of Ben's café, and a plate loaded with his home-baked (from scratch, not a bread maker or pre-mix in sight) multigrain bread, toasted just the way I like it (no burnt bits), liberally buttered and generously spread with marmalade. I immediately feel better. He heads out for his daily bike ride and I ease into another day.

I think I'm starting to learn something from all of this, to gain a sense of clarity. I can't quite articulate it fully yet, but it's to do with grace and forgiveness and letting go and being grateful and healing and kindness and self-acceptance and all of that. And only having one life. One shot. And whatever happens, I'm realising that the thing I need to do above all else is accept the cards I've been dealt and live each day as fully and as well as I can.

I thought I'd learnt all that years ago when I emerged from depression. Through reading and writing and music and travel and meditation and yoga, and taking time for myself and doing all manner of wonderful life-enhancing things, I clawed my way out of the darkness and into the light. I worked through a lot of stuff back then. I found out what matters. I made significant changes in my life. I discovered how to manage my mental health and fend off the black dog.

But then, I think I became a bit complacent, and stopped living my best life and fell back into old and destructive thought patterns, even though I kept doing all the things I love. My mind just wasn't in step.

I'm not a fan of the everything-happens-for-a-reason mindset. It's all bollocks, as far as I'm concerned. Try telling that to victims of bullying or child abuse or Holocaust survivors, or my friend who has MS, or friends whose husbands didn't survive their cancer battle, or anyone who has ever experienced any kind of trauma. But maybe, just maybe, this goddamn cancer thing is a chance to reset. Weirdly, I feel as if I'm re-discovering myself yet again. How many life-changing illnesses must I endure, I wonder, before this self-discovery malarky will be complete?

Another thought occurred to me as I walked on the beach yesterday. Maybe my purpose, maybe the positive thing I can create out of this situation, is to articulate what some people can't, or won't: to write about hard things, to express the messiness of the human experience, warts and all, depression and all, cancer and all. And to spread a little joy amongst all the messiness. For joy, I've found, is never very far away, even in the bleakest of times. All we have to do is look.

8 June 2021
Warm duvets and Allen keys

Yay! I sleep better and wake reasonably refreshed. I've never been a jump-out-of-bed-filled-with-Tigger-like-enthusiasm kind of person. Reasonably refreshed is, for me, pretty damn good. Give me a strong hot black coffee to gradually raise the refreshment level, and I can face the day. I kind of like it that way.

Among many swirling night-time visions (I'm a vivid dreamer) I dreamt that Ian and I were back in Lyon, a French city close to our hearts. We parked the car, filled with all our belongings, and wandered around looking for a crêperie. As we walked the streets, I kept worrying about the car being broken into and all our things being stolen, and no one was wearing masks, and the waitress wasn't very friendly and then I started to sneeze and felt a tickle in my throat (how can you feel that in a dream?) and *oh no, I've got COVID*, I dreamt thought, and then I woke up and realised I only have cancer (insert tongue-in-cheek emoji).

It's now a week since I finished treatment. My energy levels are definitely up since the daily slog of radiotherapy and two rounds of chemotherapy ended. When you're in it, you just have to do it, but with hindsight the magnitude of the slog becomes clearer somehow. Did I really get through the awfulness of that? How?

I spent several hours on the beach again yesterday and bathed in the ocean under winter skies. There's nothing better for the soul. I did some yoga poses and walked barefoot along the water's edge and listened to the sounds of nature and played soothing music and breathed the salty air and felt the power of the universe. It was simply awesome. Awesome is an overused word, but what I saw and felt on the beach truly filled me with awe. I'm beginning to feel more like myself again.

I never tire of the delights of living by the coast, be it spring, summer, autumn or winter. After my swim, I wrapped up warmly and gazed at the shifting sea, slate grey under brooding clouds, and thought it looked a bit sharky. Wouldn't it be ironic, I mused, à la Alanis Morrissette, if I recover from cancer only to be eaten by a shark?

In the evening I laughed long, hard and quite joyously while watching *Have You Been Paying Attention* (a comedy panel show about the weekly news for non-Australian readers – a bit like *Have I Got News for You* in the UK). Parts of it were so damn funny. There was a particular segment which made me laugh so much I almost (but not quite, thanks to years of pelvic floor exercises) lost control of my bladder. How wonderful it is to laugh from the depths of your belly. I must do it more often.

That was yesterday. This is today. Ben has gone down south with a friend for a few days, taking the dog with him. As he prepares to leave, I keep asking him if he's got this, that and the other, as if he were a teenager going on school camp rather than a 21-year-old in his final year at university. The maternal instinct, a blessing and a curse. A double-edged sword. We laugh about my mothering ways. Ben urges me to focus on myself and stop fretting about him and whether he'll be warm enough, or if he has enough dog food, or reminding him to refill Ellie's water bowl every day, or telling him where to find the new wi-fi code.

I take Ben's advice and enjoy the quiet house. It's now eight days since my last treatment. I'm in a holding period. Waiting to find out my fate. I've been doing the best job I can of living in the moment, especially these last few days. Sometimes people tell me (as if I need a reminder) that it must be so hard to wait. I don't find such observations helpful, generally. It depends who says them, and how, and with what intent, but it's not what I need to hear. I can't dwell on how hard waiting is. I prefer to look at this interim period as precious time to do the things I love, time to heal and reset and reflect. Time to be. Time to live.

That's why I mostly want to keep a low profile and do my own thing and avoid conversations and interactions that feel uncomfortable and put thoughts in my head that I'm trying to keep out.

I won't let Alan steal my joy. I won't allow cancer to break my spirit.

It's another wild, Winnie-the-Pooh type of blustery day. A typical winter's day. A bit too wild, windy and wintry even for me to brave the chilly, churning ocean. Now that I'm feeling less tired, I'm doing a bit more each day, venturing a little further from home. Trying to live as normal a life as I can. Relishing the ordinary. Embracing everyday tasks.

With the beach ruled out, I suddenly have the urge to go to IKEA. I love IKEA. Well, love is perhaps too extreme a word, but I could quite happily while away the day wandering and wondering through the maze of Swedish design efficiency, contemplating the relative benefits of the bewildering array of storage solutions. Ian would rather poke sharp sticks in his eyes. He swears that hell is a labyrinth of yellow and blue whose unfortunate residents must construct their own furniture and subsist on a diet of meatballs and raw fish.

We live a 10-minute drive away from IKEA in Perth. When we lived in England and were setting up a new home in County Durham, our nearest IKEA was in Gateshead, an hour and a half away. I never minded the drive and was always enchanted to see the iconic Angel of the North sculpture as we drove up the A1. Ian couldn't see the attraction, either of the drive through county Durham to Tyneside or shopping at IKEA or what he scathingly called "a rusty old plane that had nose-dived".

Back then, we needed a desk for the study in our new house, so off we set one fine September day. Ian lost patience after 10 minutes.

'What about this one,' I asked.

'Yes, fine, get it,' he answered.

'Or maybe this one?' I asked again.

'Sure, any of them are fine,' he fired back, his impatience growing as I continued to inspect the huge range of desk combinations on offer and request his opinion on them all.

You had to buy the table top and legs separately, which added more decisions to the process, decisions for which Ian had neither the interest nor the patience.

After what must be the shortest amount of time ever spent in an IKEA store we returned home, unloaded the goods, removed the packaging, laid out the screws and bolts and indecipherable instructions so Ian could (reluctantly) set about assembling our new desk. My husband hates DIY. He says he's no good at it. It's been a recurring dialogue in our marriage.

'You'd get better at it if you did it more,' I tell him.

'No, I wouldn't,' he says. 'It's like singing and dancing (I periodically ask him if he would like to take ballroom dancing lessons with me). I'm no good at them and never will be, so there's no point.'

'You sing and dance perfectly well after a few beers,' I tell him.

And then we argue about how anyone can do anything if they just try, and how I learnt to wield a power drill and hang pictures at just the right height, and mount spirit-level-perfect shelves, and if I can so can he.

I never get anywhere. I've even been known to say things like "call yourself a man" partly, but not totally, in jest, and compare him unfavourably to friends' husbands who can build a floor-to-ceiling wall of *Billy* bookcases before you can say Ingvar Kamprad (the founder of IKEA, for those who prefer their furniture fully assembled).

Back in County Durham, circa 1994, it took hours of muttering and cursing and unsuccessful Allen-key wielding before Ian realised we had bought the wrong legs. These days, if I buy the wrong item, or change my mind (one of the great benefits of IKEA is that you can always change your mind), I can just hop in the car and I'm there before the second song on whatever Spotify playlist I'm listening to has finished. In this instance, there was no way Ian was going to spend another "four hours of my life I'll never get back" returning to IKEA in Gateshead. It was me, of course, who did, and me who constructed the desk, which has served us well and which we still use every day. And me who subsequently undertook any household DIY tasks. (Before you accuse me of bagging my husband, Ian more than makes up for his home handyman shortcomings with his domestic prowess in every other area, so I'm not complaining.)

Unlike his father, Ben is always up for a trip to IKEA and proves a splendid helper when lugging flatpacks on and off trolleys and into the car. I don't have my helper today, but I know exactly what I want – some Kallax shelves (formerly Expedit, why the change?) and a new winter duvet. I avoid the meatballs but meander around the showroom maze quite happily, wondering if the chrome or black hanging rails would look better in our kitchen (I decide on black, but baulk at drilling into the splashback tiles and park that idea for another time), reading the ridiculous names out loud and laughing to myself. Did you know that if you spell your name backwards and put an umlaut over the first vowel, that's your IKEA furniture name? Mine is Näsus Tegdert, a flexible modular sofa range.

I get the shelving, choose a duvet, throw in an LED lightbulb and some hooks for good measure and pull into the driveway before John Mayer has finished telling me he wants to stop this train (I'm with you John, I'm with you).

Ian has left a note – he's out cycling for a couple of hours. He needs his daily fix, even in the wind and rain. In keeping with the Scandinavian theme, as the rain lashes the windows and the wind whips piles of fallen leaves around the garden and courtyard, I channel my inner Dane, light some candles, make a roasted carrot soup with cumin and coriander, rustle up a beetroot, goat's cheese, walnut and coriander salad (you can never have too much coriander), then set the table more decoratively than usual, with tealights and flowers, aiming for a Hygge kind of domestic vibe on a winter's day.

Ian appreciates the vibe and the food when he returns. I fill him in on my trip to IKEA and we reminisce and laugh about his ineptitude with spanners and hammers and drills. Which is odd, it occurs to me, given that he happily and skillfully wields a full array of cycling tools for hours on end when tinkering with his bikes in the garage.

After dinner, I rant a lot at the TV.

'You're so funny,' Ian tells me. 'Is ranting and swearing one of the side-effects of cancer treatment?' he asks. 'I didn't read that in your information booklets.'

In keeping with my ranting and swearing, I tell him in fairly explicit terms to go away. He asks if I'm channeling Nan from the Catherine Tate show.

'I hope I make it to that age,' I say, as lightly as possible, not wanting to kill the mood. 'I hope I get to be a grandmother.'

'You're actually very funny,' he continues. 'You should be on *Gogglebox*.' And we laugh some more.

It feels good to make him laugh and to sense his relief that I'm more like myself this week. I haven't given him much to be cheerful about of late.

I think the duvet may be too warm, by the way. I bought an extra warm one and sweltered through the night, probably because it was designed for icy Swedish conditions rather than Perth's mild winters. I'd have thought they'd adjust the warmth relative to the temperature of the country in question. Oh well, it only cost me $40. Pre-Alan, I'd have fretted about the purchase, buyer's regret and all that, but it doesn't bother me at all now. If it continues to be too warm, I'll donate it to a worthy cause, to someone who needs a warm duvet far more urgently than me.

9 June 2021
33,000 feet of grief

10.00 am
In 2019 I gave a presentation at the Cancer Council about mental health. Any physical illness also has a huge psychological impact.

The staff were keen to hear about my experience with depression and anxiety, learn about the signs and symptoms and find out how best to support cancer patients and their families with every aspect of their health.

I think it was one of my best presentations ever, despite my propensity to suffer from impostor syndrome. *These people are dealing with cancer, who am I to tell them what's what*, I thought at the time. I've struggled with impostor syndrome my whole life. I didn't know what it was until someone gave it a name, made it a syndrome and I read about it and thought, that's me. Never quite fit, never quite belong, never sure if I'm any good, if I'm enough.

I don't walk around doubting myself all the time, but self-doubt has always been a part of me. I've been comforted to hear and read that many creative people are similarly afflicted, including some of my favourite writers, even those, perhaps particularly those, who have become rich and famous through their craft. Most of them also happen to be women. It's not hard to work out what that tells us.

As I shook off my impostor syndrome and began speaking, the interest in the room was palpable. I had the proverbial captive audience. I could see the engagement in people's eyes, their willingness to come along for the ride as I held them in the palm of my hand. Some cried, and there was much laughter too. I've been told by people who've heard me speak that I have the ability to move people across the full spectrum of human emotion. I really don't know how that happens. It just does. They tell me it's because I'm real, I speak from the heart, I lay it all out there and my spirit shines through. Those are other people's words, not mine. I would never assume that about myself.

My mother died from ovarian cancer seven years ago. She slipped away quietly in the palliative care home to which she'd been moved just two days prior. At the moment of her passing I was suspended helplessly at 33,000 feet, somewhere between Dubai and London. My brother and sister were with her at the end. They told me it was peaceful and that she wasn't in pain.

Seven years later I don't think I'll ever fully recover from arriving too late, from not being at my mother's bedside at the end of her life. We'd spoken on the phone just before I left Perth.

'I want to see you,' she said. She knew.

Throughout her illness she never made a fuss or made me feel bad for living on the other side of the world. I'd spent time with her in the summer before she died, good, quality time. She rallied under the soft English sun after several punishing rounds of chemotherapy that worked for a while but that in the end couldn't keep the cancer at bay. During that summer we went out when she felt able, a coffee here, a lunch there, a visit to a beautiful garden. Mum loved gardens and gardening. When the summer ended and I returned to Australia, she deteriorated steadily until that grey November day when she could fight no more. I tell myself that at least I had those summer days with her, that I brought her some joy towards the end of her life, but it's never enough. I let her down. I was too late. I wasn't there at the end.

You hear about people on their death beds who hold on until their loved ones arrive, who see them, smile, utter some deep and meaningful final words and pass over to the next world. That didn't happen with me and my Mum.

Grief. It comes and goes. It's not a linear process. It still sometimes hits me so hard that I double up with such excruciating pain I can barely breathe. My father died two years before my mother, and two years before that we lost my eldest sister. All that sadness and sickness and loss were intertwined with my descent into depression and anxiety.

I've been thinking about Mum a lot, now that I know a little of what she went through. My Mum believed in God. She had a child-like unquestioning faith that sustained her through life, and that must have been a huge comfort at the end of her life. A blind faith I could never understand but that I now envy.

I don't think I believe in God or any kind of afterlife, but I won't rule him or her or eternal life out completely, just in case. If he or she exists, he or she will not be impressed with my fence sitting I'm sure, but you never know. I do see myself, however, as a spiritual person, despite my suspicions about those who profess their own deep spirituality. Such proclamations run contrary to what it means to be a spiritual being. For me, spirituality is quiet and contemplative, not loud and self-congratulatory; it means having a sense of forces far bigger than ourselves, a feeling of being part of something far greater than we can ever imagine. Maybe there's divinity in that belief.

I hope my Mum was right and I'm wrong. I hope she's having a lovely time in heaven. Wherever she is, or isn't, I've been talking to her a lot lately, telling her what's going on with me, telling her I'm sorry I wasn't there to hold her hand through all the horribleness of her cancer battle. Telling her I wish she was here, that I wish we'd been closer and had more time together. Telling her I love her.

Later

The blessed rain continues. I don't feel like doing much today. A friend calls, offering to help me become more efficient with social media and create a database and build a mailing list so I can sell more books. How kind. That's my dream, I tell her. To make a living from writing. To not have to go back to full-time teaching, much as I love it. To combine part-time teaching with dancing to the beat of my own drum. Maybe, with help from others and my own determination, I can create that life for myself. Maybe Alan is giving me a chance to do that.

So many maybes. It begins and ends with me. It's up to me to make my life happen. I realise that as I write I'm becoming more myself again, feeling much better *dans ma peau*, which seems counter intuitive given what's been going on in my body. This surely tells me something. It's up to me to listen to whatever the universe is trying to tell me. There are powerful lessons to be learnt. I need to channel the conscientious student I once was and pay careful attention to those lessons.

A friend's husband has cancer. She's been a great support, telling me she's there if ever I want to talk, or rant, but not expecting anything of me. She gets it. She gets me. We talk a little about him and me and dealing with people's questions (which sometimes feel like interrogations) and how no-one else can ever really know what someone else feels like. Fellow sufferers can, and do, certainly empathise much more, of course. But as with depression, there's no one size fits all. There are so many different types of cancer and everyone reacts differently to their diagnosis and treatment. A lucky few may sail through, but most will battle dark times along the way, even when presenting a sunny face to the world, of that I'm pretty sure.

I've never been able to do that, present a face other than one that reflects my mood, that is.

I've always been an open book, heart-on-sleeve kind of girl. This is me.

For the rest of the day, I cocoon myself, remembering what one of the nurses told me. It feels nice. The Kallax construction can wait. I read and write and snuggle up on the sofa to watch a movie on SBS. In the evening I flick between *MasterChef*, the French Open tennis and Rick Stein's *Cornwall*. The tennis is engrossing. I stay up late to watch Rafael Nadal fend off Diego Schwartzman before retreating under my very warm duvet with a new Kindle book.

10 June 2021
Shake it off

I've slept better. I must be getting used to the new Swedish-strength duvet. My friend has forwarded some links and advice to get me started after our chat yesterday, so I spend a couple of hours following up, looking at LinkedIn and connecting with a writing contact she has sent me. I need to put in the time with all of this. That's where I went wrong in the past. I was daunted by my lack of knowledge and expertise about all things digital, constantly questioned and doubted my writing ability, and allowed myself to be too easily put off. I lacked patience and persistence. I need to step up (and, while I hate the word, I need to upskill). I need to keep telling myself that I'm more than capable and can do hard things.

The rain and wind continue. Ben sends news from down south, with his characteristic 21-year-old brevity. I exercise and walk in the afternoon, undaunted by the weather, then prepare to meet a friend for dinner. It's been so long since I made any effort with my appearance, to take time deciding what to wear, to blow dry my hair, to put on makeup, a slick of lip gloss, a spritz of perfume. I've lived in pyjamas and tracksuit pants for the last few months and avoided looking in the mirror for longer than absolutely necessary, not wanting to see what Alan has done to my already aging face, to be confronted by the ravages of illness.

I sing along to Taylor Swift's *Shake It Off* as I drive to the Mount Hawthorn restaurant. It's Thursday, late night shopping, the streets are busy, and it takes a while to find somewhere to park. I feel like a hermit emerging from my cave, a prisoner released. It's exhilarating, even though inner suburban Perth is hardly New York City. The cafés, bars and restaurants hum with life, as people meet and chat and eat and drink. This is what real life is like, this is what normal, healthy people do.

My friend is waiting at our table. We keep in touch online, but we haven't seen each other for more than a year. So much has happened to us both, and to the world, since we last met. We hug warmly. I am thrilled to see her, excited to be out, to have the energy to chat to someone who understands, who knows me well, who gets the horror of cancer. My friend knows all about my battle with depression and her empathy for the cruelty, the unfairness of this new battle, after all I went through with my mental health, is deeply moving. She's had her own challenges too – aging parents, teenage children, redundancy and all the usual ups and downs of family life, the juggle, the endless juggle.

We talk throughout the meal and linger afterwards. It's just an everyday weeknight dinner, but such a delight for me.

'Try my kale,' she says. 'It's delicious. How's the fish? Shall we share a dessert? Another glass of wine?'

Buoyed by friendship, good food and intelligent conversation, I don't tire at all. We discuss writing and my hopes for what these words could become. She's a writer herself, and I'm thrilled when she offers to help in any way she can.

It's an everyday catch-up to the casual observer, but something quite magical for me. My everyday has not been anything like this in a long, long time.

11 June 2021
To the other side, and beyond

I fall asleep quickly after my night out but wake in the early hours, buzzing with creative ideas after the evening's dinner discussion. I scribble in the notebook by my bed for a while and have finally dozed off again when my phone alarm rings with cruel insistence. After several rounds on snooze mode, I can delay no longer. I need to do the usual Friday tidy-up for the cleaners. At least it forces me to get going and do something with the morning.

Tidying complete, I head to the beach with backpack, notebook, laptop, headphones and, just in case, a towel and my bathers, park the car and go for a walk. I'm tired but it's not a debilitating tiredness. I feel, in fact, quite energised and walk further than I have for a while. I'm testing out some new walking boots for the first time. However comfortable they may feel in the store, you never know how good a fit they really are until you've put new boots through their paces. I have pronating feet and need support for my weak ankles (too much hockey, multiple sprains over many years), so finding the right footwear is crucial. I start walking without giving much thought to my route and end up on a bush trail through Bold Park.

Sometimes I listen to podcasts when I walk. At other times it's music I need. Today I walk to the sound of birdsong. The clouds part and the sun beams gently down from an intense blue winter sky. Blades of grass glisten with freshly fallen raindrops. Wet leaves sparkle and dance in the sunlight. The earth smells rich and warm, the air fragrant with natural bush oils, eucalyptus, an aromatherapy air bath. Nature enfolds me in her embrace and time stands still.

When I emerge from the undulating bushland onto the coastal track, I'm astonished to realise that several hours have passed. I feel a deep sense of peace and contentment. Back at the car I pick up my towel and bathers and walk through the dunes to the beach. I get changed, run to the water and stand waist deep for a while as the waves crash and white foam forms shifting shapes and patterns around me. I lift my arms to the sky and silently give thanks for this day, this moment. I don't venture beyond the breaking waves but submerge myself joyfully until my fingers and toes begin to turn white, even though I barely register the cold.

I spend another glorious hour on the beach, stretching and moving my body in gentle yoga poses and more strenuous abdominal exercises. I relish the strength in my core and remember the resolution I made months ago, when the world turned upside down, to just keep walking. I've stuck to that commitment. I'm thrilled with my new boots and today the walk was effortless. It isn't always so. I hope with every fibre of my being that I'll be able to walk my way through to the other side of cancer, and far beyond.

In the evening I whip up a mushroom risotto and we debrief on the day and the week ahead. Ian's Dad is declining rapidly and tough decisions loom. He's been in hospital for a week. The doctors have acknowledged that Pam can no longer look after him; he cannot go home until help is in place. The burden, both emotional and physical, is crushing. Pam has been exhausted for months and facts must be faced. Ian will visit this weekend and talk to his sisters so that they can consider the way forward, which is likely to involve a move to a care home. It's such a sad time for all the family.

We clear up after dinner and watch a couple of episodes of *Unforgotten*, a British crime series with a stellar cast led by the fabulous Nicola Walker. I stay up late to watch Stefanos Tsitsipas take on Alexander Zverev in the Wimbledon semi-final. It's gripping tennis but I don't quite make the distance. My eyelids start to flutter and I fall asleep at the start of the fifth set when it looks like Zverev will triumph after losing the first two sets. I'm surprised to discover, when I wake in the night and briefly check my phone, that Tsitsipas has prevailed.

12 June 2021
Lock up your daughters

Another weekend has come around – time seems to be passing so quickly – and I prepare for my trip south tomorrow. Ben returns full of chat and a newly pierced ear.

'Parental crisis meeting needed,' jokes Ian.

We watch Ben's hockey match in the evening, a close encounter with end-to-end action throughout. His team wins after a tense final quarter. We discuss plans for tomorrow when he comes home briefly to change before heading out to a 21st party. When I ask if anyone noticed his earring, he laughs. His coach told him he used to think Ben was the only player he would trust with his daughter, but now he's not so sure.

13 June 2021
It's a beautiful day

I often watch *Insiders* and *Offsiders* on the ABC on a Sunday morning to hear some debate on the news and sport of the week. As I sit up in bed cradling my steaming coffee, I'm dispirited once again by the Australian Government's apparent inability and unwillingness to speed up and streamline our shambolic vaccination rollout (what rollout?). Add in the daily diet of mixed messages, scaremongering and seven state premiers determined to do it their way and there are far too many ego-driven fingers in the COVID pie. I'm disheartened by what seems like a widening gulf between the words and actions of our political leaders, by the endless question avoidance and meaningless soundbites that do nothing to address the needs of a country, a planet in crisis. I'm frustrated by the confusion, the nitpicking, the criticism of other states and premiers. I wonder what happened to "… we share a dream and sing with one voice … ." And silently lament that this is not the Australia I emigrated to in 1999.

In one of the most advanced countries in the world, it should be so simple: work steadily towards the percentage of fully vaccinated inhabitants that must be reached for borders to open and freedom to be regained. And, in the meantime, allow families to be reunited, without the need for quarantine, as soon as they have been fully vaccinated. Test us regularly if you must, check that vaccination is complete by all means, but at some point in the very near future please stop locking us down and locking us in and locking us out of our lives. Then we can set about living again, travelling, seeing our loved ones and leave behind this soul-sapping climate of COVID fear and uncertainty.

It's another beautiful day. I'll be heading south in a few hours to make the most of the time before my next round of appointments. Weather and body permitting, I'm planning some long walks in my new boots. I've been posting some photos on Instagram of my walk on the Camino de Santiago in 2014. It's hard to believe it was seven years ago that I trekked 152 kilometres through verdant Galician landscapes. As the pilgrim's trail wove its timeless magic,

I emerged, step by step, a little more each day, from depression, trauma and grief so deep I thought I'd lost myself.

Revisiting the past is very different from living in the past. My Camino memories remind me that even in tough times, even when facing what may seem like insurmountable challenges, there is wonder and beauty in the world. They also remind me of how far I'd come since then, until 2021 threw me a curveball, and how much I learnt back then, in the aftermath of grief and loss. I realise, also, that the lessons I learnt as I clawed my way out of trauma and depression, the changes I made in my approach to life, are just what I need right now. I vow to go back to Spain one day to walk the rest and complete my pilgrimage.

I check my phone and see that Georgia has sent a couple of photos on WhatsApp. The first is captioned "spotted" under a photo of Daniel busking in north London, some 13,000 kilometres away. It's a beautiful day over there. The sun is shining, the sky is blue, and there's a red double-decker bus in the background. A classic London sight. People are walking by with shopping bags, a few standing still as my boy sings and strums. The second is a photo of a hotel-perfect bed above the caption: "Just made up your room". I wonder when I'll get there.

My heart filled in a bittersweet kind of way, I message back and we plan to talk later today when I arrive down south. It's hot in London, she says, a steamy 28-degrees, and she's going to swim later in the Hampstead Ladies' Bathing Pond. I picture us there together two years ago, walking through the leafy streets of Highgate to Hampstead Heath in our summer dresses, passing the famous cemetery, marvelling at the elegant houses ('doesn't Sting live around here?' I asked), picking up some gourmet goodies at Gail's along the way for a post-swim picnic on the grass. Then walking around Kenwood House afterwards, remembering that scene from Notting Hill when Julia Roberts almost sabotages her chances with Hugh Grant because of an accidentally overheard conversation with a co-star.

Pre-COVID I used to jump on a plane at the drop of a hat. I'm a seasoned traveller, adept at rolling clothes into a compact suitcase, skilled at fitting toiletries of no more than 100ml into the requisite see-through bag. For flights within Europe, I'm alert to the traps of low budget airlines urging the reservation of seats, the purchase of more luggage allowance, insurance and all manner of unnecessary add-ons. Pre-COVID, I could recite the dimensions and carry-on luggage options for EasyJet and Ryan Air, and precision pack to avoid any excess charges. I once flew from London to Geneva for one pound, not including the unavoidable tax.

The roads are clear as I drive south to a soundtrack of old songs I put together this morning. Paul Kelly, Paul Brady, Nancy Griffiths. Nostalgic tunes that remind me of the early days with Ian, my first trip to Australia, the first time I drove down this road, our developing love story that spanned the globe and defied the cynics who told me that long distance relationships never work.

The winter light is fading when I arrive. I need to stretch out after the drive, so quickly unload the car and walk for an hour or so amidst the twilight kookaburra chorus, the chirrup of magpies and the rhythmic chirping of crickets. The bushland is alive with insects and creatures of the night. I catch the last of the salmon pink tinges on pillows of cloud. Small animals dart across my path. The bay is calm, the water still apart from the gentle lapping of tiny waves onto the seaweed strewn shore. The lights of Busselton twinkle in the distance and the beacons atop the posts that anchor the shark net flash orange on and off.

When I get back to the house, I call Georgia as I unpack, make up the bed and sort things out for my stay. There's a sadness in her today. It has been a stressful time, what with a house move and a new job in the same month. She's keen to hear my news. I don't want to talk too much about Alan but update her on the last week. I don't want to tempt fate, I just want to enjoy this time, this moment, relish the fact that I'm feeling good right here, right now, I tell her. I don't want to speculate about what the future may hold.

'That's a good way to be,' she tells me.

We talk about what we do to get through difficult times. We're both sensitive souls, easily bruised and hurt. I'm grateful for this friendship that blossomed over tea and Kit Kats in a London publishing house back in 1989.

What is it about tough times that makes us appreciate good times and good people so much more? Why does it take a crisis to shake us up and open our eyes to all the things that really matter? Why do we neglect to see those things when life is chugging along without incident? Why do we forget to look up and around and appreciate the bigger picture? Why do we sweat the small stuff and expend energy on people whose values don't align with ours, who dance to the beat of a very different drum? I sense a shifting within. If I get through this, I owe it to myself to choose very carefully where and with whom I direct my precious time and energy.

Our call ends and I proceed with the evening in the whisper quiet house. I'm good at being on my own, but I'm temporarily overcome by the solitude and feel suddenly quite lonely. I allow the feeling to pass through me while distracting myself with dinner and television.

Ian messages to see if I want to chat and I call straight away. He's back from the visit to his parents and plans are moving slowly towards putting sufficient care in place for Richard. He'll stay in hospital until a solution is found. There are still hoops to jump through, phone calls to be made.

I know very little about aged care in Australia, but these recent months since Richard's stroke have not filled me with confidence. The system appears messy and protracted, fragmented and derailed almost to the point of paralysis by reems of red tape and inefficiency. Horror stories about 18-month waiting lists for urgent home care packages to be put in place are depressingly common.

Despite the sadness in parts of our conversation, I'm reassured by Ian's calm understanding and acceptance of his parents' situation, as well as by his steadfast, unconditional love for me. He has a rare ability to affirm all my doubts and fears and emotions without allowing them to spiral out of control. I'm scared about next week, I confide. Really scared.

He tells me that everything I'm feeling is completely understandable. He doesn't diminish my fear by telling me not to be scared or sad, or try to fob me off with platitudes along the lines of *everything will be OK*. I love that about him.

Ian and I have never been the kind of couple that needs to be together all the time. I'm down south right now, he's in Perth, but we are as together as we have ever been. Together apart. One of the reasons we've been married for nearly 28 years is the space and time we've always given each other. It comes from a place of absolute trust. We know that together we are stronger, but we are still our own people. It's always been that way, perhaps partly because we started off in different hemispheres and found a way to be together while pursuing our own lives and careers.

Sadness, fear and the whole gamut of difficult emotions are part of the human condition and we bury them at our peril. Owning and expressing my fear about what lies ahead helps it to dissipate and gives me a renewed appreciation for this precious week.

When I'm all talked out, and we sign off for the night, I feel replenished by love. With this man by my side I sometimes feel I could move mountains.

14 June 2021
Possibilities

I wake alone but am no longer lonely as another day dawns. I've regained my equilibrium. There's a narrative of new possibilities running through my head. I've booked a Zoom call with someone I came across on LinkedIn last week. I was intrigued by her reinvention as a life coach, writer and podcaster, after leaving a teaching career that wore her down, as it does so many. She has created a successful business, part of which involves helping other teachers transition out of education or reduce their teaching load to allow space and time to explore new options. Which is exactly what I did seven years ago when I took time out to lead a more creative life and write a memoir about my journey through anxiety and depression, a book of poems and seven children's picture books.

So I know a bit about sea changes and tree changes and the desire to do something different. While I'm sceptical about the whole life-coaching industry, she was offering a free 15-minute call and I thought *why the hell not? What do I have to lose?*

Elizabeth is bright and articulate and appears very genuine, although it's hard to be completely sure in cyberspace. She's generous with her time and we chat for longer than 15 minutes. As we talk, I take stock of how much I've done and how rarely I give myself due credit. She acknowledges that I'm already some way down the path, that I've had the realisation and have the passion to lead a more creative life.

'Yes,' I say. 'I was starting to do that through writing and speaking, but it was hard to make any money.'

I'm not driven by money per se and was daunted by the mechanics of setting up and running my own business and by the minefield of technology that it necessitates. I started dipping my toes into the world of social media in a half-hearted attempt at self-promotion but found myself mostly posting pretty pictures of landscapes and pelicans rather than using it for hard-core marketing. While I loved writing and publishing my books, I barely broke even financially. I lacked the skill and knowledge, or perhaps the motivation, (or perhaps there was an element of fear – there usually is) to make any money as a sole trader. So, I backtracked into teaching as new opportunities arose in education, opportunities that were too good to turn down and that provided a steady, secure income.

I see now, with the benefit of hindsight, that I had a point to prove. I was, and am, a good teacher. I wouldn't have been able to write that back in 2013. I'd been ground down, demoralised (according to author, Doris Santoro, many teachers who think they are burnt out are actually demoralised by a system that demands more and more while giving less and less), stigmatised for disclosing my mental health battle and bullied (I didn't realise it was bullying at the time–covert, insidious, soul-destroying bullying). For the sake of my sanity, I had no choice but to resign from a job I had loved for the best part of 12 years.

It was a terrifying time. In the aftermath, as job offers poured in (much to my amazement) for replacement and part-time positions, as well as a role in examination development, I regained my faith in myself. My professional confidence as a linguist and educator was restored. It felt good.

Elizabeth ended the call with the option for a longer follow-up strategy session. I don't like the word strategy. It makes me nervous. I work on instinct, intuition, passion. But maybe strategy is what I need right now. Strategy and a proper, grown-up business plan. I no longer have a point to prove with teaching. I no longer feel like a failure.

I have a great job in a school that feels like family and I'm not ready to walk away from teaching just yet. If I get through this health crisis, I'm convinced that part-time is the way forward. If I can negotiate a reduction in my teaching load when I'm ready to return, a more varied, balanced and creative life is within my grasp. Of that I'm sure. I'm also sure that if I can attain the right balance, I will be a better teacher in my final years in the classroom. It's up to me to make this happen, to invest in myself again, to reach out and connect with people who have the know-how to help make my vision a reality.

The life coach sends a follow-up email with some links to podcasts and her website should I wish to book another call. I reply to thank her and explain that I'll need a couple of weeks to think things through. She writes back telling me she's sure I can achieve my vision without her, but it might take longer. She could be right. Having someone to make me accountable and keep me on track could make all the difference.

'The door is open when you are ready,' she says.

I get on with the day, my thoughts alive with possibility, and attempt to rein in my mind chatter (it can be exhausting) with exercise, a trip to the shops and a hair appointment. It feels so good to have the energy to do normal things. I'm exhilarated by the wild winter weather, by the squalls of rain and wind interspersed with the sudden parting of clouds to reveal the bluest of blue skies, by the sporadic bursts of sunlight. I spend the last two hours of daylight walking familiar paths along the coast, around the golf course and back through the quiet streets.

15 June 2021
This teaching (and coaching) life

I spend the morning writing and thinking. Yesterday's Zoom call continues to stir ideas and possibilities, as well as bring back memories. I do some research on Elizabeth and find that she has a series of podcasts called *Get out of Teaching*. She's a good interviewer, a clear speaker and an intelligent observer, allowing her guests to tell their stories and only interjecting to move the discussion along. I'm impressed. She has clearly established herself in this niche, having built up an international audience and solid reputation.

One episode features former teacher Gabby Stroud, who has become a spokeswoman for the growing community of demoralised teachers across Australia, and who I discovered several years ago on a Radio National interview. She's now the author of three books and is a regular contributor of articles and interviews to various media platforms. She hasn't returned to teaching, but still needs to supplement her writing income in other ways.

Another interviewee is the children's author Suzanne Gervay. She has won multiple awards and received an Order of Australia for her services to literature but makes it very clear that the creative life she leads has not been a path to riches. She found it impossible to combine teaching with her drive to write and create but hastens to add that she's no J.K. Rowling.

I understand the disenchantment with the education system - I've lived it myself to some extent – but it makes me sad. I still believe teaching is the most noble of professions. As Muriel Spark wrote in *The Prime of Miss Jean Brodie:* "The word 'education' comes from the root e from ex, out, and duco, I lead. It means a leading out. To me education is a leading out of what is already there in the pupil's soul." I believe that, and I've tried to live that. There is no better feeling than witnessing that leading out from your students' souls.

I'm not a quitter. I stepped out for a year but eventually made my way back to the classroom, dipping in and out initially, taking on replacement positions and part-time roles and then, quite suddenly, at the start of this year, finding myself in a permanent role in a school where I'd done some relief three years prior, the school with the bagpipes and rousing assemblies.

Until my health faltered, I was enjoying it immensely. My reservations about this noblest of professions remain, but I'm getting better at dealing with teaching in the 21st century with its myriad demands. At the core of it all, once you wade through the surfeit of administrative requirements, expectations, policies and protocols, the updating and feedbacking and form filling and outcoming and reflecting, it's about a lifelong love of learning and, in schools such as the one where I now work, about the strength of communities. I feel supported by the leadership team and the teachers around me, stimulated (and challenged) by the students, who teach me something new every day.

I've always loved schools. I am the daughter, granddaughter and great-granddaughter of teachers. At the age of three, I sat in the back of my mother's classroom playing with the ink pots, counting crayons and subconsciously absorbing the wonderful world of words so that by the age of four I could read and write beyond my years, like Marcel Pagnol in *la Gloire de Mon Père*. I quickly discovered the power of books and learning. Teaching is in my DNA; it courses through my veins.

People like me are attracted to teaching because we love the energy, joy and inhibition of young people, but seven years ago the education system had depleted my own joy, inhibitions and energy. Add in a mental health crisis and the feeling of being micro-managed to within an inch of my life, and something had to give.

I stepped out for a while, then eased back in, and in recent years have worked in some wonderful schools where I've felt nurtured, supported and trusted to get on with my job. The contrast with the micro-managing school was striking. When I accepted a temporary "acting" head of department role, the principal spoke more to me more in six months than the previous one had in 14 years. Going to work was a pleasure, despite the huge daily demands on the modern teacher. People looked out for each other; staff wellbeing was a priority. Tick, tick, tick.

And yet, the unequivocal fact remains that however healthy and supportive our working environment is, teachers continue to juggle multiple balls, wear many hats and play numerous roles (surrogate parent, coach, mentor, counsellor, IT expert, administration guru, first aid responder, risk assessor and accidental psychologist are just some that spring to mind) and we need to be constantly mindful of taking on too much.

No wonder teachers become good life coaches. No wonder Elizabeth was such a skilled listener. Teachers have an array of eminently transferrable skills we often take for granted. We are so bogged down with the minutiae of our daily load that we underestimate our own power.

I've done some life coaching training myself. While I was "acting" head of department, I had the opportunity to take part in a course, run by a lovely man with whom I had reconnected at St George's Cathedral (weird day – suddenly felt the urge to go to the cathedral to hear some choral music, bumped into a life coach called Michael whose daughters, we discovered, I had taught, met his wife, had an instant connection, she bought my book, we met for coffee, she told me her story; fact is stranger than fiction).

Life coaching was all the rage in schools back in 2017, when it began to take over from mentoring. I used to think that you had to wear a tracksuit and have a whistle around your neck to be a coach, but how wrong I was. Trouble is I also had a mentor at that time, as well as mentoring someone, which is different to coaching in that you give advice and pass on the wondrous wisdom you have garnered over the years.

Mentors give lots of feedback, and as a mentee – is that a word? – you receive no small amount of advice and guidance. Coaches don't give much feedback. There's a lot of sitting around in silence while the coachee wrestles with thoughts about goals and reality and options and becoming their best selves, and where to next. The idea being that a skilled coach gives you the tools to work it all out for yourself, by asking all the right questions. It's an intense (and increasingly lucrative) business.

Mentoring fellow teachers is different. Some take their role really seriously, with lots of meetings, box ticking, data entering and follow-up sessions. Others prefer to deliver their feedback over a cup of coffee and a chat, which was, thankfully, the modus operandi of my mentor at the time, wary as she was of taking up too much of the time needed to be spent aligning all the language courses and programmes with both the West Australian and national curricula, as well as mentoring my own staff.

Intrigued to learn more about coaching (we teachers are suckers for constant improvement and, much I as loathe the word, upskilling) and despite (or perhaps because of) my impaired time-poor judgement, I signed up for the six-month course.

It reminded me of the time some UK friends employed what they called an "action coach" when their business was struggling during the 2008 global financial crisis. After a few sessions, the conclusion they came to, much to my amusement, was that they most definitely could not afford an action coach. Action was swiftly taken and said coach dismissed.

I experienced something similar with the coaching course I embarked on. I withdrew from the last session because my workload was particularly heavy that week and I wanted some time to myself. Sitting in a classroom after school, albeit for worthy reasons, was not an option. A swim and a walk on the beach were needed to restore some balance.

In an earlier session, it was clear I had to prioritise time for myself. Hmm. Therein lies the irony in all these self-improving initiatives. Worthy as they are, too often we cannot find, or afford, the time to fit them in. We've become so clogged up with information that cramming one more thing into our overloaded schedules is the last thing we need.

Providing constant feedback is another time-consuming trend that shows no sign of dying down. It's all the fault of someone called John Hattie. No longer can we have a quiet word with Joel after class to suggest a few ways he might improve his reading skills. We must annotate our marks books, upload work samples and provide improvement strategies after each assessment.

And "great job, Chantelle" simply won't cut it. It's got to be something along the lines of "I really like the candid way in which you addressed the issue of drugs and alcohol, but in order to write with greater conviction and clarity, you would be advised to undertake a complete revision of verb conjugation, starting with *être* and *avoir* and moving through the verb groups systematically until you can conjugate with confidence. Only then will your very frank views on the legalisation of cannabis find clear expression."

This feedback is, supposedly, for the benefit of the unique species that is the private school parent, but as a former private school parent myself (we could only afford it because Ian's job halved the fees) all I ever wanted to know was whether my boys were trying their best and behaving themselves.

Needs must, and I have become adept at providing in-depth feedback, to which I must confess I'm often impishly tempted to add something along the lines of: "Thank you and have a lovely life, because I may never again return to teach your class, so exhausted am I by this treadmill of assessment, appraisal and feedback. So good luck, I hope your ATAR result reflects the fact that you have done absolutely no work for the past five years and have depended completely on the very large spoon I carry around with me and with which I attempt to feed your limited intellect, together with the plethora of private tutors your parents have at their significant disposal …"

The essence of the whole coaching lark is pretty sound, methinks. It would have been even better if we hadn't needed to cram our two-hour sessions into the end of a heavy teaching day. God forbid that we would get time off to undertake this training. But hey, them's the breaks of the average teacher. Take that eight-hour day and cram as much into it as possible before you return home, slump on the sofa in front of the latest mindless drivel, glass of wine in hand, then stumble to the study to input your feedback, update your professional development records, review your anaphylactic training, and then maybe, just maybe, for five minutes, when you can barely keep your eyes open, you might take a cursory glance at what you'll be teaching the next day.

At my first coaching session, I was so exhausted I gave my energy rating a two out of 10 when we had to "check in" at the start – the next lowest was a five, so I am clearly an inadequate human being with the stamina of a gnat. But I kept my mind open and quite enjoyed the exercises we were given. We had to split into groups of three at one point and talk about a time in our careers when we'd felt supported and valued in our teaching roles.

Turns out mine was in my first teaching job in the UK. Now, four years on from the coaching course, I work in a school which is paired with the school where I was first employed, through a global network called Round Square. In the twilight of my career, I am experiencing a similar level of support and validation. I have come full circle. Funny thing, life.

Did I mention that I love teaching?

One child, one teacher, one book, one pen can change the world.
~ Malala Yousafzai

16 June 2021
In the moment

After yesterday's ruminations on teaching, coaching, creativity, writing, and all manner of possibilities, I finally stepped out of the house into a mild winter's day towards the end of the afternoon. Two hours of walking; just what the doctor ordered. I ventured further along the coastal track to the solitude of Curtis Bay and spent time watching shadows lengthen and colours intensify as the clouds began their evening transformation above a sinking sun.

Then it was back home for another contented evening in my own company. I lit candles, made risotto, drank a glass of wine, chatted to Daniel and Ian. I felt certain I would sleep well but my prediction proved wrong. I spent a disturbed night, unable to reach a state of sustained deep sleep, taking refuge in my Kindle each time I stirred. I didn't feel anxious, so wonder why my slumber was fragmented. It must be the subconscious mind chatter, I tell myself now, and vow to do more of a night-time wind-down this evening: some yin yoga poses and meditation to empty the mind.

This morning, I stagger to the Nespresso machine, then check my phone while an extra strong pod infuses. Georgia has sent another photo. *Look who I bumped into while cycling on Hampstead Heath*, she writes, under a selfie of her and Daniel. My heart lurches. He looks so well and happy under the summer sun, a fresh haircut highlighting his chiseled features and dazzling smile. The London temperature has remained high and I can almost feel the heat rise up from the path and smell the freshly mown sweet summer grass in the background.

Coincidences, seemingly chance meetings, I love them. The fact that Georgia and Daniel literally bump into each other on a packed Hampstead Heath (and bump into each other for the second time in a week) on a steamy summer's day gives me a sense of forces beyond my understanding, of wonder and awe, of a universe that moves in mysterious ways. I gaze at their beaming faces and am filled with an intense yearning, a poignant joy, a surge of love so intense it takes my breath away. They are so close to me, and yet so far.

At her request, I've been sending Georgia daily photos from my walks while I'm down south. She loves the way they keep us connected. I've been sending pictures of secluded rocky coves, of evening sun piercing storm clouds to sparkle on the bay, of lengthening shadows when the coastal colours are enhanced by the exquisite evening light, of the vast mirrored expanse of water stained pink and purple by the clouds overhead.

The days are flying by. Freed from responsibility, and any routine or expectation imposed by others, I'm the closest I've been in a long time to living in the moment. I'm managing to fend off thoughts of next week, with its appointments and tests and scans, before they take hold in my mind.

It's another beautiful winter sunshine day. I get my bike from the shed and cycle along the coastal path, stopping for a quick dip at the swimming beach by the boat ramp. The air is still with barely a whisper of wind, the clear, calm water shimmering enticingly in the soft winter light. I've come prepared and find a spot by the rocks where I strip off my winter layers to my bathers. Two women chatting on a bench eye me with interest, intrigued, no doubt, by my bravery (foolishness?) as I walk towards the water.

I brace and tense and grit my teeth and mutter and yelp as I slowly submerge my whole body. It's cold, but gloriously so. Here in this still, clear bay I feel strong and alive. It's too cold to swim out to the shark net and back, or do laps parallel to the shore, as I sometimes do in warmer weather, so I just swim in and out a little, past the rocks, around patches of seaweed.

As I wrap myself in my towel, a man walking on the path above stops to commend my bravery and ask about the temperature. We chat a little. He asks if I realise the shark net isn't up, telling me that the posts are there but the net is always taken away after the summer season.

'We've had several shark sightings recently,' he tells me. 'Right by the boat ramp.'

'Crikey,' I reply, thanking him for the information but assuring him I didn't venture very far this time.

I'll stay close to shore if I swim again this week, which I plan to if the weather holds. It's too delicious to resist.

Every inch of my body tingles as I get dressed and find a comfortable place to sit on the rocks. I feel infused with life as I focus on the sound of water lapping between the rocks and gaze towards the horizon, my horizon of hope. I'm soothed by the ebb and flow, the soft swell, the timeless movement of the ocean, the winter colour palette that fills my senses.

Later, I walk on the beach for a while, further along the bay, amongst huge piles of seaweed thrown up by recent winter storms and watch the fading light and shifting colours. I never tire of this evening ritual, the dance of nature. Clouds disperse to reveal a crescent moon. It will be a clear sky night and I feel the temperature suddenly drop.

I go out with a friend for an early dinner in town. She and her husband are in the process of creating a new life for themselves in this corner of the world, having sold up in Perth in search of the sea change that many aspire to but never dare pursue. It's been six months now and she's relishing the new pace of life, the beauty of the landscape, the daily beach walks, the incandescent light, and new opportunities within this small-town community.

Back home, Ian and I chat to debrief each other on our days. Progress is being made with his Dad's care and his Mum is feeling stronger. It's good to know things are moving in the right direction.

I watch the last episode of *Bloodlands*, a crime series set in Northern Ireland against the backdrop of Belfast, Strangford Lough and the Mountains of Mourne. It stars James Nesbitt (born in my hometown of Ballymena, three years after me, so of course I know him well) as a police detective at the centre of a cold case, his craggy features perfecting the heavy-browed conflicted look. I can't quite keep up with all the nuances of the plotline (as is my wont, and Ian isn't here to enlighten me) but enjoy it nonetheless, perhaps more for the setting and the accents than the story itself. A couple of guys I used to know joined the RUC (The Royal Ulster Constabulary), now known as the PSNI (Police Service of Northern Ireland, for those who haven't see *Bloodlands* or *The Fall*), and I wonder how accurate this portrayal is. By the end I still can't work out if James Nesbitt's character was good or bad. I think the answer is that he was neither good nor bad, but flawed, as most of us are, and was forced through circumstance to make some horrific choices.

When the episode ends I do as I'd planned, and wind down more before bed with that legs-up-the-wall yoga pose that's supposed to induce sleep.

17 June 2021
Technology overload

It worked! I sleep until mid-morning, stirring a little through the night but going straight back to dreamland each time. No Kindle, podcasts or medication required. Heaven.

On waking, I spend a couple of hours writing and thinking about my social media profile, such as it is. Back in 2017 I knew I needed to market myself if I wanted to sell my books. Despite serious reservations about self-promotion, I set up a Facebook Page, an Instagram account, a LinkedIn profile and a website, with the help of people far more tech savvy than me.

Given my propensity to rant about the evils of technology I felt like a hypocrite. But I knew I couldn't beat them (whoever they are) so I had to join them: I am followed, therefore I am.

I found the sudden acquisition of a swathe of social media platforms quite overwhelming, and they still drive me crazy with their constant updates and reminders. But I discovered that if I wanted to recoup my publishing costs, get some paid speaking gigs, keep raising awareness about mental health, break down stigma, reach out to others and help them to see that they are never alone, then I needed a social media profile.

I did manage to sell some books but the paid speaking gigs didn't materialise. When COVID struck I used social media to keep in touch with friends and family through turbulent times. My feeble attempts at self-promotion took a back seat.

I'm constantly questioning the worth and integrity of social media. For a while I employed a very lovely millennial (or should that be a Gen Z-er) who helped me master (well, at least have a go at) things like Canva and stories. Which was great, but also not, in that it was a constant reminder that I am, and always will be, behind the eight ball in such matters.

I've just about worked out basic Instagram posting when I find out it's all about reels and stories now. Which aren't really stories at all, well not in my book (get it?), but merely a couple of photos with captions. And then came Tik Tok, which I gave a wide berth as it seems to be inhabited by even more narcissists than Instagram. I couldn't go there – too worried about what I'd look like, old and shrivelled as I am (what was I just saying about narcissists?). It did give me some insight, though, into the reason for the ever-decreasing attention span of today's students. Then there are "lives" and YouTube channels, pumping out supposedly purposeful content, most of which seems to rehash the wisdom of the ancient philosophers and claim it as something new.

Surprisingly, my lovely Gen Z-er was impressed with my grid (my Insta grid, that is). I wasn't quite as enthusiastic about the success of my life being reduced to, and dependent on, a sequence of small, albeit very attractive, squares, but I took the compliment with good grace.

It happened quite organically when I finally gave in and bought my first iPhone, about a decade after everyone else. My parents didn't buy a colour television until I was 14, and very reluctantly replaced our old record player – you know, those retro ones with the big lid that comes down and that are probably now worth a fortune – with a new stereo system. They never bought a VCR, let alone a CD or DVD player, so I've always been slow on the uptake when it comes to gadgets and gizmos. It's in my genes.

With my new iPhone, I started posting pictures of colourful things that caught my eye when travelling in France and Spain in those far off pre-COVID days. As I became aware I even had a grid I need to curate (which, according to die-hard Instagrammers, is a full-time job without full-time hours that brings in full-time dollars, but I've yet to master that), I started to feel the pressure to keep up appearances.

I've yet to successfully juggle and seamlessly sync Twitter, WhatsApp (where's the apostrophe?) Facebook, Instagram and LinkedIn, despite my best efforts when I log in for the modern-day equivalent of walking to the mailbox. I have fewer than five followers on Twitter; no one seemed to notice, let alone like, my handful of pathetic little tweets. I didn't really know how it worked, so I soon gave up.

And here's a question that often occupies my over-active mind. If something wonderful happens and I don't post about it, then did it actually happen? A bit like that tree falling in the woods – if no-one's there to hear it does it make a sound? Such is the whimsy of my thought patterns.

Sometimes I want the whole world wide web to come crashing down so we can all be released from the pressure to be seen, heard and liked, and go back, as Voltaire wisely counselled, to cultivating our own gardens. Sometimes I want to quit, hit control-alt-delete, never again to reboot. It can be so draining, the constant pressure to put your best face forward, exhausting to filter the mental clutter, the empty chatter, the so-called expert opinions, the need to be liked a thousand times. More like Fakebook than Facebook.

Every day I'm offered webinars and workshops that are guaranteed to help me reach my first million (followers? dollars?) within the first year if I just click and sign up now – you've always got to do it right now, so you don't miss out. There are only ever a few places left.

I can't keep up. I don't want to keep up, with the Kardashians or anyone else. It's not good for my mental health. I've felt the dopamine surge when a post receives more than the usual amount of attention (with me, that's any more than 10 views/likes and a few comments) and the disappointment when what you think is your very best original quotation, beneath your very best capture, flies way under the cyber radar. The competition can be crushing; my photo is more perfect than yours, my life more idyllic, my grid more splendid, my tweets cleverer, my stories more captivating.

And the Big Brother aspect of Facebook freaks me out. As soon as they get a whiff of the fact that you might at one time in your life have been depressed, or prone to anxiety, the cyber floodgates open and you're bombarded with mantras about the journey of life and the importance of staying positive and receive prompts to join this depression group, or that anxiety forum. Now I'm getting posts and all kinds of advice about cancer, when I haven't posted anything publicly about Alan. It's highly disconcerting.

As for all those inspirational quotations, well enough, already. Quite clearly, if I shoot for the moon, miss and land amongst the stars, I'll self-combust. And those apps that show the rain falling, or trees blowing in the wind to help us stay calm, am I the only one to think that these seem like the most damning indictment of our times? Watching rain and trees on a screen when we could be out walking through the actual rain and wind?

Despite my reservations, there seems to be no choice but to add to the noise. I'm not sure that hiding behind pictures of pelicans, coastal landscapes and scenes from your travels is the way to go, though, if you want people to know about you.

My relationship with the screens that now dominate our lives continues to rollercoaster between love and hate, with not much in between. I'm not the only one to be wary. When asked by a *New York Times* journalist if his kids loved the iPad, Steve Jobs (may he rest in peace), replied: "They haven't used it. We limit how much technology our kids use at home." Parents, take note.

I heard another great quote a couple of years ago from the comedian Fiona O'Loughlin. It went something like this: "Is there anyone out there who just goes to work, comes home, pays the bills and shuts the fuck up?" Well said, Fiona well said indeed. And the answer is, probably not.

We all do it, don't we? Very few of us "shut the fuck up". We get sucked into thinking the world needs to hear our opinion, fooled into believing that we are "liked" therefore we are. Maybe sometimes all we need to do is "shut the fuck up" – once we've had our say of course – put our feet up and watch a bit of TV, old style. I may just do that one of these fine days.

It would be such a relief to have the courage to opt out.

I'll continue to post the odd photograph and pen the occasional reflection to share with whomever happens to be there at the time. Because things move on so quickly in the virtual world. There's no point agonizing about whether your post is perfect enough because after just a few seconds, if the algorithms don't pick it up, it will be the cyber equivalent of the discarded newspaper that wrapped your fish and chips once upon a time.

Facebook is quick to send alerts if I haven't posted anything for a while, urging me to boost my posts and reach more people. Which reminds me that I did once put a couple of faces to Facebook. On our last trip overseas, Ian and I signed up for a Spanish cooking class in a gypsy cave in Sacromonte (Insta-heaven) and in our little group were two very gorgeous young women from California. We got chatting and found out they worked for Facebook. After several copas of sangria I was telling them all about my forays into social media, waxing lyrical (while Ian talked to a very nice, quiet Kiwi group member and pretended he didn't know me), asking their advice and no doubt boring them senseless when they would much rather have been flirting with the very attractive chef or learning more about Andalusian culture and cooking.

But they were nothing but delightful. I told them I received regular alerts from Facebook telling me they hadn't heard from me for a while, and that I wanted to get more followers to my page but didn't really know how to get my social media shit together.

'That's me, that's what I do,' said one of the women. 'It's my job to track the pages and the algorithms and send out alerts to get people to post more.'

'Oh my God,' I exclaimed in my mildly intoxicated state, thrilled to be having this behind-the-scenes-at-Facebook encounter. 'That's amazing, I can't believe that's you!'

Meeting someone who worked for Facebook hasn't enhanced my profile one bit, but now when I get those alerts, I think of that beautiful young woman sitting in some uber trendy office in Silicon Valley (is that where Facebook HQ is?) working her cyber magic, even though she probably moved on long ago to work on a start-up for the next big thing.

One day I might just forget all about hashtags and handles and herd goats on a Tuscan hillside for the rest of my life, but until then I'll continue to dabble on the fringes of the virtual merry-go-round.

On the positive side, whenever I feel like I'm losing my mind and becoming a little forgetful, up pops Facebook to tell me what my memories are. Thanks, Mr Zuckerberg.

Late afternoon
The power of nature

I have a sudden urge to drive to Yallingup. I love the contrast between the sheltered tranquility of Geographe Bay and the wildness of the ocean on the other side of the Cape. It's that wildness I now crave. There's something in the air that tells me that's where I need to go; I listen to my intuition.

I park at Caves House and walk along the Ghost Trail, through the gardens and valley, alongside the brook to the little town. Then down onto the magnificent beach, a pristine sweep of sand that curves towards the granite formations of Cape Naturaliste, extending past Sugar Loaf rock and around the headland beyond, a primeval stretch of landscape relentlessly pounded year-round by massive Indian Ocean swells. I walk as far as I can northwards, until the sand comes to an abrupt end against the rocky outcrop.

The rolling surf is majestic beneath the setting sun. I sit for a while. Huge waves crest and hover before thundering towards the shore in a crashing, powerful symphony of nature's glory. Sea spray dances in the golden light, lifted high by the ebb and flow of the surging mass of water. I'm at one with the elements, energised by the roaring ocean, my spirit infused with the pure, clear air as I marvel at the timeless forces of nature. I feel connected to my inner wildness.

I sometimes wonder if what the world is suffering from is nature deficit disorder. I defy anyone to walk along this beach and not rise above all the pettiness of humankind, not experience that "peace which passeth understanding" and a sense of wonder. It could, it should, be so simple. Nature gives us perspective and sanctuary from troubled times.

Mine was a childhood of open fields waiting to be explored; of long summer days on the spectacular Antrim coast; of headlands and coves, harbours and rockpools, windswept beaches and towering cliffs; of peaceful glens, mountain streams and secret waterfalls; of hedgerows bursting with blackberries ripe for picking when September came; of bowls of strawberries fresh from my father's allotment, devoured with lashings of cream and sugar, an early summer treat made so much more special by the shortness of the season; of lazy afternoons shelling peas in the back garden; of winter days tobogganing, then tramping home for mugs of hot chocolate by the fire; of enchanted walks through woods and forests, looking for leprechauns and faery folk; of whizzing down country lanes on my bicycle. A childhood spent connected to nature.

The south-west of Western Australia reminds me of my childhood. That's why I feel so at home here. The vegetation is different, the climate warmer, but the essence, the feel, the spirit of this small corner of the world fills me with a sense of belonging and connection for which I'm especially grateful now.

Still deep in contemplation, I walk back along the beach and up some steps to a viewpoint where I survey the shoreline and catch the last of the sun's rays before making my way back to the hotel carpark.

Caves House is like something from an Agatha Christie novel, the perfect setting for a classic murder mystery. The barman did it on the Rose Terrace with his cocktail shaker. I've always been captivated by the unique atmosphere of the heritage-listed house and gardens, the roaring but hidden ocean a constant background accompaniment. The carefully tended gardens, filled with secret corners for lovers' trysts and hidden nooks for all manner of dastardly assignations, appear to tumble effortlessly down the hillside.

Murder mysteries aside, the house has a colonial, art-deco vibe reminiscent of a Somerset Maugham short story, with its terraces, bay windows, high teas and lounge bar. I walk through the ground floor of the hotel, instead of around the side, to soak up some of this atmosphere. People have clearly dressed for dinner. There's a roaring fire and a piano and double bass duo plays classic tunes. I savour the moment, briefly imagining myself in a stunning gown and long gloves, smoking a cigarette through an elegant holder, hair perfectly coiffed, lips Chanel red. I blink and, suddenly conscious of my sandy boots and windswept appearance, continue through the bar and back to my car.

It's dark when I get home. I light candles and listen to music and make dinner. I'm alone but not lonely. Later, I chat with Ian and watch the *Friends Reunion*. Ben has watched every series so many times he can recite the dialogue of each episode word for word. I message him to compare notes. We're both sad that Matthew Perry is clearly not in a great place. A salutary tale about the trappings of fame and money not being the key to happiness, we note. We debate and joke about the amount of "work" Courteney Cox and Jennifer Aniston have had and agree that Lisa Kudrow looks the most natural of the three women, although we love them all.

Ben then tells me he's put my Kallax shelves together – he's always up for a spot of Allen key action. I'm delighted.

I fall asleep replenished by love and an afternoon spent in nature.

All this ancient wildness
That we don't understand. ~ Snow Patrol, Life on Earth

18 June 2021
Three months on

9.00 am
I'm grumpy this morning. I thought I'd cracked the sleep thing, but restful slumber was elusive last night. I have no idea why. I wasn't thinking about anything in particular.

I resolve to shake off my grumpiness and get on with the day. I note that it's exactly three months since my diagnosis but I'm feeling pretty good and I'm not going to let anything burst my south-west bubble. I listen to John Mayer as I drink my coffee, the volume and caffeine hit cranked up to enhance my mood. There's stormy weather on the way but, for now, it's another day of sun (anyone else love *La La Land?*).

11.00 am

I'm not grumpy anymore. I will cycle and swim and walk and all will be well.

19 June 2021

Apron strings and maternal pride

In need of a solid night's sleep, I resort to over-the-counter medication and wake in the late morning, feeling groggy but pleased to have slept for at least ten hours. There's a cold front passing through, bringing wind and rain and a drop in temperature. Undaunted by the weather, I cycle into town to buy a newspaper in the morning and walk in the afternoon, stopping off for a quick plunge in the turbulent water along the way. As always, it's worth the cold hit for the warm and tingly afterglow.

In the evening I chat to Daniel. He's in a reflective mood, looking back on all he has seen, done and learnt during his four years in London. From renting a room no bigger than a cupboard, to months of couch-surfing, relying on the kindness of friends and often not knowing where he would be sleeping from one day to the next, he finally found a place to call home. I think about those uncertain years now, and I shudder; he was, quite literally, homeless for six months.

He talks about the things he has learnt about himself and what makes him happy. He's less of an introvert than he thought. While, like me, he needs time on his own to recharge, he enjoys having people around and thrives on friendship and conversation. We weren't designed to live alone. He has the perfect balance now – space when he needs it and company when that is what he craves.

I think about Daniel for some time after our chat. About how proud I am of this young man who seems to have far more worked out at 24 than I have at 58. About how hard he has worked and continues to work to make his way in the music industry, to find out whether he can make an acceptable living from his craft. I'm trying to step back, to avoid offering too much advice, to loosen the virtual apron strings that tie me to this beautiful soul, to understand that he needs to do life his own way.

But I worry about him and his future. In a world where extremes flourish and the ability to shock attracts most attention, I wonder what chance he stands. He doesn't have that Harry Styles woke way with fashion, innate confidence and awareness of his own sex appeal. He's a typical shorts and T-shirt Aussie-British boy. He has no tattoos or piercings and doesn't wear make-up or jewelry. He's not a rebel with or without a cause. He's been thinking about his image and wondering how to revamp his online persona. But would it ultimately serve him well to pretend to be something he isn't?

20 June 2021
Write what cannot be said

The wind and rain rage through the night, in and out of my dreams. In the vivid, visual territory of strange dream content, I'm back at university trying to find somewhere to live; I discover

I'm pregnant while preparing for my final exams (an event that didn't happen, by the way). Then I'm dream-walking through the streets of Leeds with all my worldly goods in a plastic bag (another event that, thankfully, didn't ever happen).

Here and now, back in the reality of the winter of 2021, it's my last day in the south-west for the time being. The week has surpassed expectations. I've nourished my body with good food and my soul with the things I love. I've walked and cycled and exercised every day and felt connected to nature. I've listened to my favourite music, made new playlists and discovered new podcasts. I've curled up to read books and articles and watched gripping TV shows and entertaining films in a candlelit room.

I think back to how I dug myself out of depression seven years ago, learnt to manage my mental health and live a full and joyful life again. I discovered so much about myself in that chapter of my story. Those discoveries continue to sustain me now.

Any physical challenge can have a huge impact on mental health – the incidence of depression and anxiety has soared in this COVID era – and I'm grateful for the knowledge I now have, through my lived experience and work with Beyond Blue. I was determined to create something positive from my journey through depression and anxiety. I wrote what I could not say, and in doing so found the courage to speak up. Writing this new story has brought me to the same conclusion. Whatever lies ahead, I am determined to create something positive from the curveball I was thrown back in March.

Why does it take a life-threatening illness for me to do the thing I love, I wonder? Whatever happens, I need to make writing part of my daily routine and stop making excuses – wrong chair, wrong desk, no room of my own, too much noise, not enough time. I'm fabulous at excuses. No more.

I remind myself again that in 2017 I published nine books by attending workshops, sourcing editors and designers and typesetters and liaising with all kinds of people to bring my projects to fruition. It took months of emails back and forward and proof-reading and more proof-reading, and after all that there were still a few typos, godammit. But now that I'm a proof-reading fiend I keep picking up errors in other books, so I mustn't beat myself up too much.

My picture books have been popular in schools and libraries, even though I wasn't aiming for the educational market. I remember writing the first one in my head along the Camino in 2014, and marvel at how a simple idea became a reality. A teacher friend made me smile last week when she told me a student of hers had chosen one of my books during their library session.

Excuses notwithstanding, I have kept writing, albeit rather sporadically, since then. I had an article published in the *Weekend Australian* travel section a couple of years ago, and one in the *Review* section a couple of years before that. That's two articles submitted and two published. Two from two. Not bad (but no paycheck, sadly). And then there are the blogs on my website. They're more like articles but I'm told it's better to call them blogs, that the word "article" sounds too serious and might put people off. I find the whole blog thing interesting, and not just a little confusing. I write a blog and I'm immediately given feedback from my friendly website host (I think that's the name of the thing that gives me the feedback) telling me my sentences and paragraphs are too long, I don't have enough keywords interspersed throughout my text, my slug is too short/long and there's something wrong with my SEO.

Excuse me, I want to say if anyone was listening, I learnt to read and write long before the internet was a twinkle in Bill Gates' eye, before algorithm was even a word. I was a straight A student in English language and literature, and you are telling me how to write? In the words of Catherine Tate (or one of her many alter egos): How dare you. How very dare you.

Short sentences, short paragraphs, small attention span, small brain. What's happening to the language of Austen and the Brontes, of Shakespeare and Trollope and Dickens? I don't think those literary giants would have taken kindly to such correction or given a stuff about slugs and SEOs.

I jest (or maybe not so much). Writing keeps me sane. Most of the time. It can also drive me crazy. I have numerous notebooks filled with ideas and jottings and remembering what I wrote and where I wrote it is quite a feat. Ideas come to me in the night, or in the middle of doing something else, and if I don't write them down then they can just disappear into the ether as quickly as they came into my head and, try as I might, I can't bring them back, they've gone, floated away on the breeze. This happens to Elizabeth Gilbert too, by the way, so I'm in good company. And the fear thing, too. That's part of the whole writer's angst to which many attest, Marian Keyes being a case in point. Fear of failure, fear of not being good enough. It has to stop.

I can shake off everything as I write; my sorrows disappear, my courage is reborn. ~ Anne Frank

21 June 2021
Hope

I'll be heading home soon. Tomorrow I have appointments with Charles and Tony. I have no idea what the next couple of weeks will bring. It's been so nice to write about things other than medical procedures. I'm hoping for the best but trying not to speculate too much.

I keep checking in with my mental state to make sure I'm not depressed. I'm worried and anxious, but I know depression well, and this is not it. Over the last week I've felt as much joy and awe and wonder and connection with the universe as I ever have.

They say that depression is the absence of hope. I'm quietly hopeful about both my health crisis and my writing future, given the progress I've made in the last couple of months. With writing, hope can very easily lead to flights of fancy that keep me amused and distracted from cold, hard reality, something that surely cannot be a bad thing in the current circumstances. Here's some proof that hope (delusion?) plays a big part in my life, a common scenario I like to re-run in my head. It goes something like this:

Receive message from Reece Witherspoon (who discovered me through my spectacular Instagram grid) telling me she's buying the rights to my book and will be casting herself and Matt Damon in the leading roles – well, I'm actually the leading role so Matt Damon will be in the supporting role of my long suffering husband, for which he (Matt Damon, not my husband) will be nominated for an Oscar, but which he won't win because in that year (possibly 2024) Christian Bale will win the Oscar for his portrayal of Donald Trump and the atrocities of his inglorious presidency, impeachment, fraud, fake news, crimes against Mexicans et al.

Ben would prefer Jennifer Aniston to play me but, much as I adore Jen, it's Reece all the way for me, even though "the Rachel" was my go-to haircut throughout the nineties. Sorry Jennifer, but *Wild*, *Big Little Lies* and *Little Fires Everywhere* cemented Reece as my pick, despite her sickeningly perfect, envy-inducing Instagram grid (with which she has, no doubt, more than just a little bit of help).

See, I live in constant hope … oh, and there's more. My mind is a fountain of hope these days. Lisa Millar invites me onto Breakfast@yourabc to talk about the film adaptation of my previously little-known book, and how it's likely to catapult me into all-time stardom given Reece's (and Matt's, albeit supporting) patronage and asks how it feels to be just an ordinary person from Perth who has reached out, spoken up and done what she can to reduce stigma and break down barriers surrounding common mental health conditions such as anxiety and depression, and less common cancers such as Alan.

'Well, Lisa, I'm humbled, of course, but it feels great, it feels FUCKING great,' I reply.

'I'm sorry Sue,' Michael Rowland interjects while Nate gives the weather report. 'But could you curb the expletives, this is a family show after all.'

'Of course, Michael,' I say, duly chastened. 'I will endeavour to curb my potty mouth, but please don't judge me … didn't you know that the judicious use of swear words is a sign of intelligence?'

You get the picture. I'm abrim with hope. I could go on ad infinitum. Following my stint on breakfast@yourabc, Lisa is so taken with my engaging personality, sparkling wit and insightful commentary that she calls her BFF Leigh Sales who interviews me on *7.30* the following night and we all swap contact details and set up our own private WhatsApp group.

A little while later, following the critical success of my film, interviewers are queueing up to get me on their show and I fulfil a lifelong dream to sit on Graham Norton's couch, alongside the stars of my film. And Bradley Cooper because, why not? Better still, I get to pull the lever on the big red chair and eject someone trying to tell a frankly very dull story about erectile disfunction.

Hope (or grand delusion) does indeed spring eternal in my crazy, over-active mind. Better crazy and over-active than numb and lifeless.

Hope never abandons you, you abandon it. ~ George Weinberg

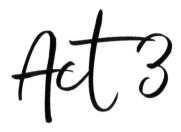

22 June 2021
Back to reality

First up, backside check with Charles. After a long and lovely sleep, I don't feel too anxious as I drive the familiar route to the hospital. I remember my first appointment, and the aftermath of shock and blind terror, and realise how far I have come. I resolve to channel my inner Marcus Aurelius and react to whatever I find out today with stoic-like acceptance. I'm still filled with the joy and wonder of my week away and feel an unexpected sense of peace.

I've sat in so many waiting rooms during the last few months. At the start of all this, I'd be jumpy and twitchy, unable to settle to anything, annoyed at being made to wait, worried about what I would find out and fearful about my future. Today I've come prepared, both mentally and practically. Specialist doctors rarely run on time. They often get called away for emergency surgery or a patient crisis that needs immediate attention. Rather than feeling indignant and impatient about delays, I've finally worked out that the best approach is to expect to wait for at least an hour. That way, anything less is a bonus.

Equipped with notebook, Kindle and headphones, and my phone loaded with playlists and podcasts, today I am the most patient patient ever in the history of follow-up cancer checks. I'm all over this waiting lark.

The reception area is bright and spacious. There's a huge floor-to-ceiling window framing a group of trees swaying in the breeze against a blue-sky background. I watch the moving picture for a few minutes, then take out my Kindle. I'm just getting to a critical scene when the receptionist calls me in. I'm momentarily tempted to tell her Charles will have to wait while I finish the chapter. That's how damn cool I am today. Cool, for me, is a rare occurrence so I want to relish it.

I take a seat opposite the surgeon and respond to his questions about how I am and how I found the treatment. He makes notes and explains that this is just a preliminary check, and that three weeks post-treatment is still quite early, but he'll have a look at the area. We go into an adjoining room where I lie sideways on the bed and pull down my clothing so he can conduct the inspection. I'm apprehensive, but not too anxious.

'It's very good,' says Charles, following his perusal of my rear end.

He then elaborates on what he means by "very good," explaining that he'll do a more thorough check in three months, and that I'll have regular scans for the next five years. But what he says he sees, or doesn't see, makes me cautiously optimistic about Alan's demise.

I get dressed and we chat some more. He's clearly pleased. I have more follow-up appointments next week with Greg and Simon, the radiotherapy and chemotherapy oncologists, and this afternoon's appointment with Tony, the ENT specialist, to further discuss the separate matter of the inconclusive throat scans and biopsy.

When the consultation ends I thank Charles profusely, choking back tears. As I walk through the hospital and out into the crisp winter air I allow them to flow, knowing that I've come through something huge and the signs are good. I'm moving in the right direction. But I can't get ahead of myself. I don't feel like popping the champagne just yet. A favourite word comes into my mind: equanimity. I repeat my mantras: one day at a time; just keep walking.

I do just that to get to the next appointment. It takes about an hour, which is exactly the time I have to spare, through Subiaco, down Rokeby Road, then along Kings Park to Hollywood Medical Centre. I set myself up in the reception area. This time the wait is longer, but I barely register the delay.

The ENT receptionist is an acquaintance and Facebook friend of mine. When I first came here, trembling with fear and anxiety, it was nice to see a familiar face. Daniel and her son were at school together and we chat about our boys. She's seen photos of Daniel online and comments on how grown-up he looks, "like a real man". She says that her boy still has a baby face and shows me a photo. I have a sudden memory of the two of them running side by side in a pre-primary sports carnival.

When Tony eventually appears, he asks if I mind a student doctor accompanying him.

'No problem,' I say, and chat to the student about his studies and medical ambitions.

Tony tells me the student is one of the best he's ever had, before spraying the foul-tasting anaesthetic up my nose and threading a camera down each nostril. This is the fourth time I've had this procedure and I take it all in my stride.

'COVID tests will be a breeze by comparison,' I tell Tony, and he laughs.

He views the pictures afterwards on his computer, then puts his fingers down the side of my tongue and throat for a rummage around. Not fun either, but I'm unperturbed. The model patient.

The upshot of it all is that Tony still thinks the best next step is a full biopsy, and another scan, which we book in for a month hence.

'Hopefully to rule out, rather than discover, anything nasty,' he says, adding that there is no need to do it any earlier.

I'll need to apply my newfound mental strength to this one and do all I can to put it aside until the time comes.

I message Ian with an update and suggest we go out for an early dinner. His Dad has come up to Perth today for a heart operation and Ian will visit him after school. He responds to my cautiously optimistic news with a row of emojis.

I retrace my route back to the car. I could go a more direct way, but I like walking through Kings Park, the towering trees and bushland of one of the world's biggest inner city green spaces a reminder of the universal timelessness of the natural world. In Subiaco, I stop off to buy soufra again and browse in the bookshop before settling on *The Scholar* by Dervla McTiernan, a crime thriller that has won numerous awards. McTiernan is an Irish author who now lives here in Western Australia; I'm keen to see if the book lives up to the glowing reviews. At the checkout, I'm delighted to discover I still have credit on my loyalty card and only have to pay four dollars.

7.00 pm

Ian and I debrief on our respective days over pizza, tacos, salad and a glass of wine at a local restaurant, buzzing with week-night chatter.

'We should do this more often,' we say simultaneously, clinking glasses and laughing.

Ian's Dad has just come out of surgery and is still very groggy. He'll stay in hospital in Perth for a couple of days before being transferred closer to home. The future is uncertain beyond that, but the hope is that by next week a care plan will be in place that will allow him to leave hospital. Ian thinks it unlikely his Dad will be able to return home long term, now that it's clear Pam can no longer carry the burden of the around-the-clock care he needs.

We discuss the school holidays. We'll head south to Dunsborough together for a week, and then perhaps move on to Denmark, depending on whether our tentative plans to visit friends work out.

26 June 2021
Getting into the Stoics

10.30 am
It's been a tough week for Ian. His Dad has been stranded in hospital in Perth since his operation on Tuesday. The plan for an immediate transfer back to Peel was thwarted due to a lack of beds. Pam has stayed at home and Ian has taken time off school to help his Dad endure the frustration of waiting; the hospital here is not set up for post-operative care and recovery.

Richard is putting on as brave a face as possible, but the situation is clearly taking its toll. Pam is waiting at home, fretting about the uncertainty and delay. Ian is spending the best part of each day in hospital, while desperately needing a holiday and wanting to spend more time with me now that term has ended, but also wanting to do the right thing by his parents. He feels completely torn in two.

Ian seldom takes time off work and has more than a year's worth of unused sick leave accrued. His conscientious nature is commendable, but sometimes I wish he weren't quite so dedicated. Instead of delegating and asking someone else to sort out his classes in his absence, he stays up late and gets up early to send detailed lesson plans (for up to seven lessons each day) to avoid any disruption to his students' learning.

I know how rare this is, and unless you are a teacher yourself you won't have any idea of the workload involved. When I worked as a relief teacher, lesson notes rarely contained much more than instructions to continue an investigation or prepare for an assessment. Often, there were no guidelines at all, and I had to make up a lesson on the spot.

Ian will never leave someone else to sort his work out. That's just not how he rolls. He goes about his business without fanfare, getting little or no thanks or acknowledgement, I fear, for his meticulous attention to detail and concern for his students' learning. I hope they know how lucky they are to have him as their physics teacher.

When I returned from down south, I stayed in my bubble of tranquility for a while but as the week progressed anxiety crept back in, a nagging agitation stirred by watching Ian rushing from pillar to post, his commitment beyond the call of duty to his work and the uncertainly surrounding his parents' future. I'm deeply saddened by Richard's situation, but also unsettled, mindful of my own health and the need to sustain my equilibrium so I can continue to rest and recover. Is that selfish? I remember the nurses' advice about cocooning and putting myself first but find that hard when there's so much else going on.

And then I feel guilty for wanting to focus on myself. Am I a bad person for resenting the impact on my own welfare and desperately wanting Ian to have a break after what has been an extremely intense term for him? Am I a bad person because I want us to have some time to ourselves, without the burden of looking after aging parents, at least for a while? Am I selfish for wanting to spend this holiday time with my husband?

I've been getting into the Stoics lately, in the hope that their age-old wisdom will help me stay mentally strong. I remember my stoic-like approach to Tuesday's appointments and try to tap into this mindset again, before I spiral into further resentment. It simply does no good to focus on the fairness or unfairness of any circumstance.

The Meditations of Marcus Aurelius was one of my father's favourite philosophical texts and my mother used to tell me how stoically Dad bore all his ailments. I thought being stoic meant you couldn't show your emotions, that you had to bottle everything inside, grin, bear, and always maintain a stiff upper lip. There wasn't much emotional language in our family, no comforting dialogue to be had through tough times, scant consolation through the turbulent years of adolescence.

From what I've read, stoicism isn't like that at all. It's not about the suppression of negative emotion, it's not numbing yourself to the inevitable troubles of life, but rather finding the courage to accept every part of being human, including difficult emotions. The key is to learn how to speak and act reasonably in the face of those emotions.

I'm no scholar of philosophy but, for what it's worth, here's a little of what I have gleaned from my limited reading. Stoicism does not mean we need to suppress our tears and resist the need to cry, which is, after all, the body's natural response to stress. The damage caused when we don't express our sadness, because of some erroneous idea that we mustn't cry, can be catastrophic. Feelings of sadness and pain are important and need to be acknowledged. The stoic approach means that by striving to see the world rationally when we cry, we'll avoid being swamped by despair, sadness and pain when those natural emotions arise.

The fact that the word stoic evokes a lack of emotion for the average person does this philosophy a great injustice. Rather than propose a passive, sweep-it-all-under-the-carpet approach to pain and suffering, stoicism offers a blueprint for the pursuit of wisdom, perseverance and the quest for self-mastery through the acknowledgement and acceptance of pain. It is not some nebulous philosophical stance, but rather a way of living based on taking action and shifting our thoughts so that we can approach life more wholeheartedly.

Given that wholeheartedness is a buzz word favoured by modern-day gurus such as Brené Brown, I would suggest that stoicism is at the core of much of the life coaching and Insta-philosophising of our age.

According to stoicism, things and events don't cause us most trouble, but rather our perception of them. It identifies the four cardinal virtues as self-control, courage, justice and wisdom. It's up to us to choose how we respond and use our reason in the face of external events. Stoicism proposes ways to counter the unpredictability of daily life by mastering our perceptions, decisions and actions and accepting the things we cannot change through clear judgement and an understanding of our place in the world. Such mastery will lead to the mental clarity we need to lead effective lives and deal with whatever comes our way.

If only it were that simple. These are the things I need right now: mastery, mental clarity and clear judgement. Ian has just messaged and there's no prospect of his Dad being transferred today. Pam will now drive up to Perth. Ian is at the helm of his family, communicating with his sisters on the other side of the country, comforting and caring for both his parents. I pray (to whom I don't quite know) that we'll all be imbued with the spirit of Seneca and Marcus Aurelius and that we'll find the mental clarity we need to get through all this.

My agitation hasn't been helped by not writing every day to help untangle and navigate my emotions. I must be disciplined and persist. When I was down south, it flowed so naturally. I had the luxury of space and time. Now that I'm back home, amidst the turmoil of the current situation, it takes greater persistence and discipline to recreate that space and time.

1.30 pm

On a more positive note, I've managed to keep walking, exercising and connecting with nature throughout the week. I've watched furnace-orange sunsets in the afterglow of swims in the winter-cold ocean, walked coastal tracks and tramped through bushland in the rain and wind. I've still found room for joy and wonder despite the constant anxiety that gnaws away in the background.

The other day I had coffee with a friend of a friend, a woman who's been through cancer and now helps other cancer survivors transition into a new field of work or adapt their existing careers in the aftermath of their illness. I warmed to her immediately. We sensed the kindred spirit in each other and promised to keep in touch.

We talked about wake-up calls and finding balance. I told my new friend that I thought I'd had my mid-life health scare when depression struck. I thought I'd been dealt my short straw, only to discover that I'd drawn another one at the start of this year. I told her about how and why I started writing, and of the challenges I faced in the aftermath of depression. We spoke of workplaces and how they can affect us, about covert bullying and narcissists and how disappointing it is to be treated badly by our own sex. About how so many people are affected by such treatment, and how so few speak out for fear of retribution. About how bullies are adept at making the other person seem like the wrong doer. About how we both created something positive out of difficult situations and will continue to do so in the aftermath of our cancers. The world needs more people like my new friend Louise.

Later

I spend a few hours at the beach and regain some equanimity. Ian has just arrived home when I return. There is still no sign of a transfer from Perth to Peel, still no beds available, but Richard is bearing up as well as he can. Pam was able to drive up to visit him and Ian reports that she seems stronger and he feels more relaxed.

After dinner we continue watching *The Undoing* with Nicole Kidman and Hugh Grant, enjoying the sense of escape into the gripping drama, someone else's drama. Ben comes back a while later with some friends and we briefly talk about their evening and what we're watching. The girls say how "hot" Hugh is and they watch *Love Actually* in the other room. Their exuberance and laughter fill the house. Ian heads to bed after episode five.

'It's too intense,' he says.

He needs time to process it before watching the conclusion. I stay up to binge to the end, which doesn't disappoint.

I then chat with Ben and the girls. We talk about actors and the movie world. Ben told the girls about the time we met Emma Thompson. We once holidayed at the same resort as Emma and her family. Ben was 10 then and made friends with her daughter in the kids' club, unaware of who she was until one day he found out his new friend's mother was *Nanny McPhee*.

Emma was a delight – cropped hair, no makeup, no fuss; just another mother on holiday. There's much squealing and excitement about all this (and much reprimanding of Ben for losing touch with Emma's daughter) and even more when we tell them that my friend's actress daughter's actress friend (who is good friends with Daniel) went out with Tom Holland (*Spiderman*) for a while and that Daniel was once on a FaceTime call with all of them. We don't really know any of these people, they are not part of our lives, but this friend of a friend of a friend chat is harmless, escapist fun and it's good to end the day with laughter.

This is life and life will go on.

27 June 2021

In search of clarity

I find a message from Georgia on my phone with two photos when I wake up. I see a young couple, glowing with vitality. In the background are hay bales and green fields and dry-stone walls, with a tree-lined hillside beyond. The woman is heavily pregnant. In the first photograph the couple is arm-in-arm, cheek-to-cheek, the man holding the woman tightly against him. Both are smiling, their joy and love for each other palpable. In the second photograph they have turned sideways, the man proudly cradling the woman's swollen belly as their smiles turn to laughter. It takes me a moment, just a fraction of a second, to process that the couple is us, Ian and me. The baby in my belly is Daniel.

It was the summer of 1996, and we were living in the north-east of England, close to the Durham and North Yorkshire border, in beautiful Teesdale, excited about the imminent birth of our first child. When I show Ian the photographs we marvel at our youthful looks, remember our happiness and something shifts within me. I feel yesterday's anxiety abate as calm and clarity take its place.

Feelings fascinate me. Who knows why at one moment we feel agitated and at another we can feel quite calm, without any obvious rhyme or reason, no matter what is going on around us. Why, sometimes, when everything appears to be going smoothly, we have a nagging sense of unrest, while in the face of obstacles we can become an ocean of tranquility. Is it because we become suspicious when everything is going well, wondering how long it can last, whereas when problems arise it's as if we knew all along they would happen, and are ready to tackle them with stoic resolve? Maybe.

Guilt intrigues me. The deep depression I went through was compounded by an almost crippling sense of guilt. I didn't deserve to be depressed. I had a good life. I was ungrateful for what I had. I was a privileged, well-educated, middle-class woman and I needed to get over myself. So much harsh judgement and negative self-talk. I wouldn't say such things to my worst enemy, so why say them to myself?

Now that I've been through cancer treatment, I find myself comparing my lot with others once again. I've only had two rounds of chemotherapy (and am praying I won't need more) while many people endure it for months, even years. I found my tumour early; many people don't. Having paid years of private health premiums, I could be treated in very nice private hospitals. I had enough money in the bank to pay the very expensive (despite the Medicare rebate) radiotherapy fees. Not everyone does.

The bottom line in all of this is, I think, that there is no hierarchy of suffering, that we should resist the urge to compare our struggles with others. If you're experiencing sickness or sadness or trauma or depression or anxiety, it doesn't matter what the cause of that pain is. It's your pain and it matters, whoever you are and whatever your situation.

Telling ourselves we don't deserve to feel the way we do is a futile and dangerous exercise. What causes untold anxiety to one person might be a minor inconvenience to someone else, and vice versa. We're all just doing our best to get through on any given day. We need to allow ourselves the freedom to express our struggles, from the minor to the major, from missing a bus to receiving a cancer diagnosis; doing so helps us keep them in perspective.

Experts and researchers have written at length on the topic of comparative suffering. Brené Brown spoke recently of this unhealthy phenomenon in relation to the pandemic. She commented that: "fear and scarcity immediately trigger comparison, and even pain and hurt are not immune to being assessed and ranked. My husband died and that grief is worse than your grief over an empty nest. I'm not allowed to feel disappointed about being passed over for a promotion when my friend just found out that his wife has cancer … the refugee in Syria doesn't benefit more if you conserve your kindness only for her and withhold it from your neighbour who's going through a divorce."

The damage caused by comparative suffering works both ways; it's equally detrimental whether we see ourselves as suffering too much compared to others, or as undeserving because other people's suffering is far greater than ours. If we indulge in such comparisons, our mental health can quickly deteriorate. We may become resentful and bitter, experience guilt and unworthiness, lose perspective and ultimately experience burnout, anxiety and depression.

I've been through the whole gamut, from a (thankfully shortlived) *why me, it's not fair* reaction to my cancer diagnosis, to feeling guilty that there are many others worse off than me. It's a challenge to keep things in perspective, to care for myself while still having empathy and compassion for others. What I learnt during my recovery from depression has helped me maintain some perspective on suffering and manage the unhealthy thoughts and comparisons that inevitably arise.

OK. Therapy session over. Maybe I'm onto something. This self-analysis could save me a fortune.

> *Although the world is full of suffering, it is full also of the overcoming of it.* ~ Helen Keller

28 June 2021
A timely escape

I wake in a tangle of bedding after one of those frustrating travel dreams where everything goes wrong. In this one, I'd been on a coach to catch a ferry from Larne (in Northern Ireland) to Cairnryan (in Scotland) and when the driver unloaded all the luggage, my two cases weren't there. The rest of the group I was travelling with, a collection of friends and family I couldn't name now but seemed so vivid in the dream, carried on with the ferry journey, leaving me on my own to sort it all out. Then I found myself flying to France, having retrieved one item of luggage, the one containing my passport, and sleeping in a shared backpacker dormitory somewhere in Nice, and it pouring with rain, and trying to contact my French friends but forgetting the code to unlock my phone and feeling stranded and desperate and then I woke up! Horrible.

Reality is not so horrible: we are heading south later today, and I start to think about packing up again. We originally planned to leave tomorrow, Tuesday, as I had another follow-up appointment scheduled, this time with Greg, my radiotherapy oncologist, but the clinic calls to tell me the appointment will now be by phone due to new COVID restrictions, enforced because one person has tested positive. One person. I message Ian to suggest we leave tonight. No lockdown has been announced, just restrictions, but the Premier is looking tense in press conferences and it's making me nervous. Ian agrees that we'll leave this evening.

I've barely unpacked from my solo trip so it doesn't take long to get ready. Mid-morning, I drive on autopilot to the hospital to see Simon for the first time in six weeks. He has received the encouraging report from Charles, and my "very good" blood test results from last week. He uses words like "disappeared" and "cured", words I find hard to accept because I know there's more investigation to come at the end of the month in another area of my body.

'Even if that investigation uncovers something nasty, all will be well in the end,' Simon says reassuringly. I think he really believes that, so I must too.

We talk some more about my ongoing recovery from treatment and how the pain I felt towards the end abated fairly quickly, more than in most cases it would seem. I need at some point to give myself credit for all of this, to feel proud of the way I coped with everything and my determination to stay active and as strong as my body would allow, to recognise that I'm now in recovery. Ian and I will have lunch at our favourite winery down south, I decide, and raise a quiet glass in acknowledgement.

While I'm at the hospital, Ian sees our financial advisor to go through the implications of my six months without income, and uncertain future income, before visiting his Dad, who's still in hospital but feeling a lot stronger. I usually fret about all things financial, but I'm uncharacteristically relaxed. I'm beginning to accept that, as everyone has been telling me for the last four months, my health must come first. I stop off on the way home to walk along a beach track and through some bushland. It's warmer today, but windy, the ocean wild and foaming as befits the season.

We spend the rest of the day preparing for our trip, talking to Ben, checking dates and explaining we may be away for three weeks, depending on whether or not we make it to Denmark. I want to make sure he'll look after the house and the dog (*of course I will, Mum, go and enjoy your holiday, I'll be absolutely fine*) before we leave. Ben then goes off to play his floorball grand final, Ian packs the car expertly around his bike, I do my usual OCD checking of whether I have everything, and finally we can leave.

We're about 50 kilometres away from Bunbury when Ben calls to ask where we are. I panic for a moment, wondering if something has happened to him.

'There's no problem,' he tells us, 'But the Premier has just announced a four-day lockdown for Perth and Peel, with effect from midnight tonight.' .

We've just passed through the Peel region with two hours to spare before the roads will be locked. First of all, phew. We escaped just in time for a much-needed getaway for Ian after weeks of juggling work and me and his parents' predicament. He's borne it all with good humour most of the time, but it's been a real slog. I would've been really upset (and forgotten all my stoic resolve) if our holiday had been sabotaged, and am so thankful for the appointment change and our decision to leave tonight.

But secondly, WTF? How long are we going to be held hostage by this virus? Other countries are moving on and the UK will soon open up fully, while here in Australia we're lagging behind the rest of the world with our appalling (embarrassing) inefficiency surrounding vaccination, mixed messaging and reliance on what now seem like archaic lockdowns and hotel quarantining.

This morning, Simon confirmed it was safe for me to proceed with vaccination. So, I called the closest medical centre, the one where I got my finger stitched up, and they told me they didn't yet know if they'd get the Pfizer vaccine, for which I'm now eligible due to a change in the age cut-off. I would've happily had the Astra Zeneca, by the way, but can't because of this rule change.

'We should find out more at the end of the month when the government makes further announcements,' said the receptionist.

Why is it taking such a long time for us to be able to book in for vaccination? People hesitating will be put off even more by the inefficiency and confusion, giving the anti-vaxxers more time to spread fear and misinformation and delay the chance of a return to some semblance of normality.

I rant a bit about all of this as we drive. It's so unsettling. Ian agrees.

'But at least we're here, on our way south,' he says. 'We need to focus on that and enjoy it.'

He's right, of course. We have no control over government decisions. It's hard, though, having no idea when we'll see our son, when he can return to Australia or we can fly to him.

It's late when we arrive in Dunsborough. We unpack, eat, watch a bit of the Tour de France and Wimbledon. All is well in our little down south world.

29 June
Marriage musings

I sleep well, putting aside all thoughts of vaccines and lockdowns, and wake refreshed. It's been a stormy night. There's another windswept south-west day happening outside and I'm keen to get me some of it.

Today's walk takes me through four seasons in a few hours. Sunshine, showers, wind from all directions, calm ocean, then stormy ocean and a rainbow. I optimistically take bathers and a towel but when I get to the swimming beach the water doesn't appeal. It's a churned up, murky, browny-green sort of colour, and full of seaweed. I opt to walk the last stretch home barefoot along the beach instead.

While walking is my thing, cycling has been Ian's exercise of choice since he stopped running. It's not quite a case of never-the-twain-shall-meet, but Ian thinks nothing of a speedy 70 kilometres on the bike before breakfast and I could never keep up. On top of which, a pre-dawn wake-up call goes against my natural body clock. Since he stopped running, Ian needs his daily fix on two wheels to stay fit in body and mind. In recent months, as he juggled his parents' needs, caring for me and the ever-increasing demands of teaching, he has needed it more than ever to clear his head and retain his sanity.

In the evening, we have a smorgasbord of sport for entertainment: The Tour de France, Wimbledon and the European Football Championships. I've always loved watching football and am a staunch England supporter, despite the frequent disappointments, missed opportunities and traumatic penalty shoot-outs they put us through. Tonight it's a classic, England v Germany. Can England break the curse they've carried since 1966 and finally win at Wembley? Can they avoid another heartbreaking penalty shoot-out? Will manager Gareth Southgate finally get some consolation for the misery of his own missed penalty against Germany in 1996?

Ian and I love watching and playing sport. Our relationship started with a game of badminton after a brazen bet that I would win. Ian's a talented tennis player and coach but had never before played badminton, whereas I grew up hitting shuttlecocks. How hard could it be? I lost the bet, and we took it to the pub.

Romance blossomed over pub lunches, more games of badminton (revenge eluded me) and squash, which was also new to Ian. I smugly won our squash matches initially – I played in the Essex premier league after all – but once he'd worked out how to use the walls and I'd taught him everything I knew, there was no stopping him. We played tennis, too, which I thought I was pretty good at until I saw Ian's textbook perfect ground strokes and crisp volleys. He was in another league entirely, but we had a lot of fun in those early days, long before we realised that a boy from Perth and a girl from Northern Ireland might just be a life match made in heaven.

Ian was my rock as I battled my way through depression and he has been my rock once again this year. No marriage is perfect, though, and like most people we've had our ups and downs.

In the aftermath of my depression, it became clear we were going through the midlife stage when many marriages come unstuck. Several of my friends were walking away from conjugal cohabiting that no longer met their needs. I was both amused and concerned by a quote I read about gay marriage just before the vote in 2019: "Of course I'm going to vote YES. Gay people have just as much right to be miserable as the rest of us."

We were by no means miserable but, like any couple, we've had our moments. This year has helped me appreciate what being married really means, how precious it is to have someone love you unconditionally and care for you with unwavering love and devotion. I'm so damn lucky. How could I ever have questioned our marriage, I now wonder. Doesn't everyone at some point, though, question their relationship and look back to sliding door moments?

Being married to the same person for a lifetime is quite a feat and I am sure we're not alone in going through a transitional stage in the last few years. Rather than raise an eyebrow at the divorce statistics, I think it's a bloody miracle that so many couples stay married. People change. People's needs change. Sex drives diminish. Once endearing habits become annoying mannerisms. Ambitions shift. For a marriage to stay healthy, it must evolve. And people often resist change, fear evolution and want everything to stay just how it always used to be. And that's an impossible wish.

I'm not someone who sees separation and divorce as a failure if the relationship has run its course. When I was in the grip of depression there were times when I wondered if maybe a 25-year stint with two amazing offspring was the best we could hope for, and maybe we simply needed to be grateful for that and move on. It's a huge achievement to stay with one person for over 20 years, and bear their children. No-one can ever take that away from you.

Independent adult children: how dare they grow up and stop gluing us together as we pick up and drop off and encourage and comfort and counsel and nourish. What to do without that glue? We need to find a new type of glue in our empty nests and through our advancing years. Maybe one with fewer adhesive properties, but something firmly binding nonetheless.

As I moved through recovery from depression and realised I'd not just survived but was beginning to thrive, I wondered whether our paths were diverging rather more than was healthy.

True to stereotype, when Ian reached his half century he discovered the joys of cycling and morphed into a MAMIL, a middle-aged man in lycra (I would be a MADIM: a middle-aged dame in meltdown). But not for him, a gentle Sunday pedal down the coast to Fremantle and back. He'd be up at some unearthly hour for a swift 80 kilometres before work, thank you very much. Meanwhile I'd languish in bed, struggling to summon up the energy to stumble to the kettle, resenting his irritating morning chirpiness.

It felt a bit like being married to Lance Armstrong without the drugs. Unless he has a stash somewhere I don't know about. As well as the activity itself, being a cyclist seems to involve much ordering of parts and accessories online, the subsequent delivery of myriad packages containing all manner of gear and gizmos to enhance life on two wheels, and hours tinkering with the bike in the garage.

Ian's new obsession highlighted our physical differences. Apart from our body clocks being wired completely differently, Ian seemed to be going through some weird age-reversing process and honing his body into a rock-hard, fat-free sculpted thing that was making me increasingly conscious of my middle-aged softness. Unlike his, my body had started to slow down; walks had become more sedate, yoga gentler, visits to the gym a rarity.

By the start of 2019 I knew I had to do something about my rapidly expanding waistline. I didn't enjoy feeling slow and sluggish and was sheepish about my lack of form beside my hubby's age-defying conditioning. So, I got back on the bike, so to speak, returned to the gym, started walking more regularly, acquired a set of hand weights for home workouts, began to think more about what and how much I ate, cut down on the wine (and Tyrell's chips, a weakness of mine) and slowly began to shed a few kilos.

I enjoyed my new routine. After the first few weeks, daily exercise and healthy eating no longer became a chore but simply part of my life.

I've kept it up, and at the start of this year was fitter and trimmer than I'd been in a long time. I felt younger, lighter, faster, better. And then came Alan.

At the time, I wondered how cancer could strike someone who appeared to be fit and healthy. I was fit, but clearly not healthy.

Perhaps being fit has helped me through these months and will continue to help me recover and get through this anus (sic) horribilis.

Back to my lycra-loving husband. Everyone knows that couples need common ground, shared interests. Ian and I also need time and space for ourselves, and I'm convinced that our space and time giving is one of the main reasons we've lasted so long. But as cycling became such a focus in Ian's life I began wondering about the common ground. It wasn't that I resented it in any way, quite the opposite in fact. It was just that our six-year age difference (he is the younger) was becoming more apparent and I felt he might be leaving me behind.

Throughout these transitional years we did a lot of travelling, which always brought us closer again. We seemed to get on best when we were travelling. I found myself longing for the school holidays when we'd head to the UK or Spain, or France or Italy. In our daily lives, all we seemed to talk about was household organisation. *Who's doing the shopping, what's for dinner, who's making it, where's Ben, how's Daniel, who's taking which car?* All reassuringly mundane. No major scandals. No double life with a mistress in an adjacent suburb. That really happened to someone I know. Another kicked her husband out; he moved round the corner and they've remained on friendly terms. Yet another reached the limit of her patience with her spouse's excessive drinking and snoring and has set herself up in a nice little townhouse near the river. One left the family home without a word of warning while her husband was enjoying his long service leave in Europe.

When Ian had long service leave in 2018 he spent five months cycling around France, Italy and Switzerland. I gave him a huge send-off with a surprise party for his 50th birthday. God knows how I kept it a secret. There were so many clues in the final days, but he missed them all: the fridge stocked with enough food to feed an army, cartons of wine arriving, new playlists labelled "Ian's 50th" appearing on our premium family Spotify account … observation has never been his strong point. He was well and truly blindsided when he arrived home from golf (another great invention for giving me space and time) and everyone jumped out of the darkness yelling "surprise", just like in the movies. I've always wanted that to happen to me, but I reckon making it happen for someone else is just as good.

Then off he went, into the sunset, bike secured in a special (very expensive) travel bag, accessories and lycra lovingly packed in a bewildering number of pouches of all shapes and sizes, professional standard bike shoes, the works. I flew back and forward a couple of times to ease the pain of separation. Although I rather liked the time on my own, which worried me somewhat, and Ian was too busy counting kilometres and scaling the peaks of the Tour de France to miss me, but I guess being on your own temporarily is very different to facing a future of endless solitude.

Much has happened since then, and our transition to the next stage of our lives is going pretty well. Towards the end of 2019 I figured I'd never beat Ian, but I'd quite like to join him, so I revamped my gym routine to incorporate longer stints on the bike. The goal being that I would be able to cycle with him during a trip to Spain in January 2020, just before COVID changed the world. As we now know, the virus was already out there, but we were blissfully oblivious to what lay ahead as we pedalled through the spectacular Sierra Nevada. I matched Ian on every climb, even passing him on some ascents, returning for more the next morning feeling refreshed and rested, without a single ache or pain in my body.

Electric bikes are wonderful things.

Post-COVID and post-Alan, I'm looking forward to many more motor-assisted cycling adventures with Ian. We've found the perfect formula.

> *Let there be spaces in your togetherness and let the winds of the heavens dance between you. Love one another but make not a bond of love: Let it rather be a moving sea between the shores of your souls.*
> ~ Khalil Gibran, The Prophet

30 June 2021
A festival of sport

England did it! We watch the match highlights in the morning. Three lions, two goals, no penalties, simply awesome. I jump around the room as Wembley Stadium erupts when each goal is scored. We laugh at Gary Lineker and his fellow presenters dancing with joy in the commentary box. If you aren't into European football this will mean nothing, but for a girl who grew up watching *Match of the Day*; who wrote an English O-level essay about going to her first live EPL (before it was called EPL) match at Stamford Bridge; who saw the great Manchester United team of the 1980s play Spurs at Old Trafford, Bryan Robson, Mark Hughes, Glenn Hoddle, Ray Clemence et al; it was thrilling.

The last time Ian and I watched England play was in a bar in France during the 2018 World Cup. They lost to Croatia in the semi-final, in one of those heart-wrenching matches that got away. I was so sure they were going to win. My disappointment knew no bounds, much to the amusement of the bar clientele. Devastated as I was (devastation being a relative term, you understand), it was fun to be in France when the French became world champions a couple of weeks later.

Celebrations over, we catch up on the Wimbledon news. Wimbledon, The Euros, The Tour de France, it's a festival of sport. Roger Federer has scraped through to the next round after his opponent, who was ahead in the match, had to retire injured. Nick Kyrios's five-match thriller had to be suspended. Everyone seems to be slipping and falling over. There is some criticism of the courts. But it's Wimbledon, the grass in the green and pleasant land is perfectly mown, and it's happening as Britain emerges from an eternity of restrictions and lockdowns. On the first day I was moved to tears when the crowd responded with tumultuous applause as the female scientist who led the team that created the much-maligned Astra Zeneca vaccine was announced as a special guest on Centre Court. A poignant moment. Get vaccinated, people of Australia. #vaxournation

I love Wimbledon. It's in my blood. I used to spend the two weeks of the tournament glued to the television when I was growing up and would hit tennis balls against the garage door for hours on end, pretending I was Evonne Goolagong.

My 2021 tennis hero is cancer survivor Carla Suarez-Navarro, who lost to Ash Barty in the first round. She only finished her treatment, which included eight rounds of chemotherapy (as opposed to my two rounds), in January and was declared cancer free six weeks ago. I watch her post match interview, in both English and Spanish, and marvel at her spirit and grace. I'm uplifted and inspired by this amazing human. Power to us all.

There has been a lot of falling over in the Tour de France, too. The police are looking for the woman who held up the sign that caused a major crash, many injuries and several withdrawals. We wonder whether cycling is now a clean sport after all the doping scandals. Ian is doubtful, but I'm a trusting soul and like to think so. We started watching the *Lance* documentary before we came down south and now pick up where we left off. Ian can't stand Lance Armstrong. Not because he doped, but because he lied about it for so long and because he is a bully. He had him picked out as a drug cheat years ago, after his first Tour victory, when the rest of the world was bedazzled by his achievements, not the least of which was fighting and beating Stage 4 cancer.

I watch the first episode of the documentary with new interest in this controversial figure as he describes his diagnosis with testicular cancer in his early twenties, his determination to survive and the gruelling treatment schedule. I can't help but admire his life force and be inspired by his survival story. Ian understands why it gives me strength and hope, but he still doesn't like Lance and what he calls his socio-narcissistic personality.

We debate this some more, in a good-natured way, before going about the rest of our day, walking, swimming, cycling. On my walk I listen to the latest Brené Brown *Unlocking Us* podcast about her book *The Gifts of Imperfection*. Today it's about cultivating self-compassion and authenticity and letting go of perfection and what other people think of you. It resonates strongly.

In the evening we go out to dinner, a spontaneous decision. We need to celebrate, says Ian. I'm not sure I'm ready to celebrate anything just yet. It makes me nervous when we clink glasses. I don't want to jinx anything. I still have a scan and a biopsy to come. I'm still in limbo. The meal is nice, but I'm unsettled. I've been keeping my head down, trying to focus on the moment, to take one day at a time, to walk my way slowly through this invasion of my body, to learn how to handle this curveball I was thrown back in March. Step by step, moment by moment, day by day serves me best. I'm not counting any chickens just yet.

1 July 2021
A kindred spirit

I feel the need to reset, to find my way back to my down south bubble. When Ian goes for his ride mid-morning I savour the quiet house for a while, then listen to John Mayer at full volume as I do my weights and stretching. It feels good. A little later I cycle along the path to my swimming spot and feel refreshed after a quick dip. It's chilly but the water is calm today and the sun warms my body afterwards. I find a spot on the rocks and sit for a while in contemplation, listening to the waves, the timeless ebb and flow, gazing out to the horizon, bringing it all back to my breath, my core. Just breathe and be, I tell myself.

I lock up the bike and start walking, without really thinking where I'm going. I find myself on the track to Castle Bay and keep walking. When I get to Castle Rock, I have a crystal clear, almost painful, memory of Daniel climbing to the top of the rock when he was four. I can feel the same anxiety I felt back then, the terror that he would fall over the edge into the sea. But I can also see my beautiful, smiling little boy and feel immense gratitude for the love of nature and sense of adventure that his childhood instilled in him.

We spent many happy family holidays in this corner of the world, long summer days building sandcastles and crabbing and swimming and kayaking and walking the coastal tracks. As I stand looking up at the rock and out to sea a woman appears, as if from nowhere, and asks if I'm a local.

'Semi-local,' I say. 'I come here a lot.'

'I love this track,' she says. 'It's my spiritual home. I want my ashes to be scattered right here.'

We talk some more, and she tells me she moved down from Perth a few years ago. I tell her about my boys and their childhood holidays and how much I love it here, too. It seems like the most natural thing in the world, this conversation with a stranger.

My fellow walker carries on in the other direction, but suddenly reappears when I get to the Castle Bay car park.

'I must tell you about the quendas,' she says. 'I've been seeing lots of them. You need to look to the side of the path. They look a bit like bandicoots.'

She tells me more about the local wildlife and where to find an osprey nest with a newborn and we both marvel at how lucky we are to be right here right now. It's a perfect moment in time. Without saying anything, I know that we recognise the kindred spirit in each other.

I experienced encounters just like this on the Camino, beautiful conversations with complete strangers along that sacred trail. Some lines from a hymn spring to mind: "We are pilgrims on a journey and companions on the road, we are here to help each other walk the mile and bear the load." You don't need to believe in God to see the wisdom and beauty in those words.

I give silent thanks for this day and continue my journey, my load a little lighter.

2 July 2021
From unease to peace

I have an unsettled night and stay in bed for most of the morning, not sleeping, but reading, writing, thinking, listening to music, trying to find my way back to my best self, to shed the irrational worries that have crept back in recent days. I reflect on Brené

Brown's podcast, reread extracts from a book on stoicism and start to feel a bit better.

When Ian gets back from his ride, I initiate a conversation about how I've been feeling but it doesn't go well. He misunderstands what I'm trying to say, feels disappointed, I think, because in his mind we've been having a wonderful time, which we have. I feel frustrated because I can't clearly articulate what I want to tell him. I can't quite work out what it is myself, so how can I express it to someone else? Not wanting to get upset, I decide to go for a long walk and ask Ian to pick me up later at Meelup beach.

As I walk, I try to untie the knot of emotions tangled up inside me. I know I need to be gentle with myself. Rather than analyse why I'm so on edge, I should just accept it in the knowledge that it will pass. The steady rhythm of walking is relaxing, as always. I remind myself I've been on a rollercoaster ride and that any feelings of unease are not just normal but to be expected.

I mentally track the last four months: the shock of diagnosis, the fear and disbelief; being told my cancer can be treated and hasn't spread, only to be told a few days later that there's something else in the scans that looks suspicious, but that it can't be investigated until the initial problem has been dealt with; the daily slog, the brutality of the treatment; the soul-sapping fatigue; the relief of coming out the other end; the waiting to find out if the treatment has worked; being told it has indeed worked but not quite being able to believe that; a period of absolute grace when I had my mini-retreat; the ongoing recovery from treatment that I'm living right now; the weeks of waiting for the next scan and biopsy.

The narrow coastal path holds me in its soothing embrace. I walk to the soundtrack of nature. The path follows the coastline through an expanse of natural bush, shaded and woody in parts, exposed and rocky in others. The sea surges back and forth on my right. The wind blows through my hair. Above me is a shifting canvas of clear blue sky, white streaks of cloud on the horizon, layers of grey above and higher up, to my left, towards the setting sun, brooding iron-grey storm clouds loom large, threatening rain.

When I arrive at my destination, I see a woman wrapped in a towel on the beach, watching her two boys in the surf with their boogie boards. As the sun moves behind the cape, the pink and orange hues from the canopy of clouds is reflected in the swirling sea. It's hypnotic. I have my bathers and towel in my backpack but I'm feeling so toasty warm after my walk that I can't quite garner the will to strip off and brave the cold.

As if sensing my hesitation, the woman walks towards me and I ask how the water is.

'It's wonderful,' she says. 'It's nature at its best.'

Two minutes later I'm rolling in the surf as the pink and orange hues deepen above and all around me and for a few blessed minutes I'm at peace.

Ian is waiting in the carpark. We drive back to town, stop at the shops, head home, make dinner, watch some more of *Lance*, then the Tour de France. We speak a little about our earlier conversation. I tell him that all is well but sometimes, on some days, I need to retreat inside myself for a while, and sometimes I feel guilty about that and start to question everything and feel my mind spiralling.

'I'll always give you time, you should know that by now,' he says.

And I do. I do know that. This man has my back and always will. And it's normal that he sometimes gets exasperated or frustrated when I can't match his mood. He has his own mind and his own thoughts to deal with and process.

Before I go to bed an Instagram post pops up on my phone from Brené Brown. She writes this: "… authenticity is not something we have or don't have. It's a practice, a conscious choice of how we want to be … there is no authenticity without boundaries. This is tough for those of us who were raised to believe that being liked and keeping people comfortable are more important than our own self-worth or self-respect."

I love and need this evening food for thought. Thanks, Brené.

3 July 2021
Companions on the road

There's a cold front on the way. Today may be the last of the fine weather for a while. We make the most of it and do a loop walk around Yallingup, starting at Caves House, then passing Ngilgi Cave before a slow climb to the top of the ridge and a spectacular descent. It's nice to have my companion with me on the road today.

Ian and I used to walk together a lot. Our first holiday was walking in the Derbyshire Peak District. We spent our honeymoon camping and hiking in Scotland and many subsequent holidays trekking in France. When we lived on the Yorkshire and Durham border there were spectacular walks stretching from our front door in all directions, across moors and down dales.

Now, in Yallingup, we sit on a bench to admire the view and eat the rolls I prepared earlier. They taste amazing; food always tastes better outdoors. As usual, I have my towel and bathers in my backpack and can't resist going down the steep steps to the beach for a swim while Ian phones his parents. Afterwards, we walk back along the Ghost Trail to Caves House, making up stories about murder mysteries and bodies hidden in the beautiful gardens. Back in Dunsborough we stop off at a little bistro for an aperitif, Spanish style, a glass of wine and a plate of jamón serrano. Just perfect.

For dinner, we devour steaming bowls of pasta with bolognaise sauce and freshly grated parmesan and open a bottle of red before watching *Dream Gardens* on ABC. I'm no gardener but I love gardens. Ours has been in dire need of attention for some time. It's my dream to have a beautiful garden, to gaze through the expanse of windows we installed during our renovation so we could view our future picture-perfect garden. It hasn't happened yet and I'm beginning to lose hope that it ever will.

Ian and Ben do bits and pieces to keep it tidy, but it doesn't look good, and I periodically threaten to bring in a landscaper at great expense. I even told Ben recently, only partly in jest, I'm ashamed to say, that he should contact one of those shows that does garden makeovers for special people and tell them his mother is recovering from cancer, his Dad is exhausted from juggling everything – me, ageing parents, imparting knowledge to reluctant adolescents – and could they please send a team of gardeners to work their magic and surprise us with our very own dream garden.

I tell Ian about this as we watch a patch of barren land transform into a verdant paradise.

'Come on Ian,' I say. 'There have to be some perks to having cancer. I'm sure that very nice English gardener who's on one of those shows, Charlie something, would love to make my day and speed up my recovery with his wondrous way with all things green.'

And we laugh, a lot, and make up scenarios and sob stories to tug the heartstrings.

Ian hates all that reality TV stuff when contestants cry on *MasterChef* and *Survivor* about missing their family, grieving loved ones, or overcoming serious illness. He finds it contrived and manipulative. Me, I love it. And actually, I now point out to him, our story is real, my cancer diagnosis was real, it's not a sob story. And it might just win me my dream garden, if only a member of my family would write to Channel 10 or 7.

No matter. It's been a Saturday of simple pleasures. A very lovely day.

4 July 2021
Great expectations

We watch the highlights of England's quarter final against Ukraine when we get up, without checking the result first. I feel ridiculously nervous but needn't have worried. It's a consummate performance. England dominate from the outset, score four spectacular goals and concede none. Wow. I can't quite believe the result. I'm far more used to sitting on the edge of my seat as they defend a narrow lead, only to concede a late equalising goal, then continue the stalemate through extra time before losing on penalties.

It's American Independence Day, and my sister's birthday. She's 68. I send her a message on WhatsApp to let her know there's a card on the way. My family are big on birthday cards. My Mum always used to remind me to send cards to my siblings and would admonish me if I forgot.

My sister replies to my message, lets me know the card has not yet arrived and then tells me who is seeing whom and doing what and where and when. I feel like a terrible person for resenting the fact that she can see both her children and her grandchild while we seem interminably separated from Daniel. Can't I just be happy for my sister for god's sake?

I try to take Taylor Swift's advice and shake it off. It's a wild, wet and windy day. The rain has set in for the rest of the week. Ian braves the roads on his bike while I potter about at home, pop into town for a few provisions and prepare another hearty winter-warming dinner. Later, we walk together again, this time from home, along the coastal path to the start of the bush trail. I tell Ian how I've been feeling about my family, how my sister's birthday has brought up old issues. He listens patiently. He understands.

'What would Seneca say,' I ask, and we laugh.

It's become something of a catchphrase, now that we've both been reading about the stoics: *What would Seneca/Marcus Aurelius say?*

'He would say that you cannot control anyone else's actions,' Ian tells me, as I nod in agreement. 'That you've done your part, sent your sister a card and messaged her, and that having any expectations of how she will or should respond is a futile exercise.'

He's right, of course.

'I'd just like her to acknowledge how hard it is for me to be separated from Daniel for so long, to recognise the pain of separation, to ask how I'm coping,' I tell him, even though I know the stoics are right and I should have no expectations whatsoever.

A quote from the *Simpsons* comes to mind again: "Expect the worst and you'll never be disappointed." Perhaps the stoics would change it to "expect nothing" rather than the resoundingly negative "expect the worst".

Ian knows how vulnerable I am when it comes to my siblings and understands my need to protect myself from further hurt at this tough time, to avoid exposure to painful feelings, to conserve my energy and focus on healing and recovery, not on old wounds. I think back to what the nurses said about dealing with people, about choosing your team, your tribe, the people who know you best, who accept you as you are and love you unconditionally, those you trust to nurture you and walk beside you through stormy weather. Ian gently advises me, again, to tell my brother and sister about what I've been going through and is certain they would send their love and support from the other side of the world.

The walk fills me up. The wind has died down. I'm enchanted by the changing evening light, the shifting reflections in the gently rippling water as we walk and talk. Nature enfolds me in her embrace once more. I breathe deeply, survey the scene and am restored. I need to preserve moods like this, moments like these. I know just how transient they can be.

7 July 2021
A change of plan

The stormy weather has set in for the week. The wind blows relentlessly and violent squalls of rain pound the roof throughout the day and night. I'm invigorated by the ever-shifting moods of the bay on my daily walks, and marvel when shafts of sunlight briefly pierce through dark grey clouds to bounce off the ocean.

We've had a quiet couple of days. Yesterday we curled up for the afternoon with books and TV and chatted about our garden. Ian even drew out a plan of what it might look like; there's hope on the horizon.

We'll be going home tomorrow. The friends we were going to visit had to change plans because of lockdowns across the country affecting their family business. We're all at the mercy of this goddamn pandemic until enough of the population get vaccinated.

On Monday I set up my VaccinateWA account and tried to make a booking online for my first jab, but there must have been some glitch in the system. It was one of those frustrating online experiences where you go round in circles and nothing works. No wonder people aren't getting vaccinated when the booking process is not only so protracted – create an account, complete various stages, answer questions about your health and ethnicity, give consent, blah blah blah – but faulty. Such inefficiency won't help persuade the hesitators should they venture onto the government site. My blood was boiling so much I had to have a cold shower, followed by a plunge in the chilly ocean in between squalls of rain to calm down.

We drive into Busselton for lunch in the bistro that serves the best crêpes I've had outside France. Thibault, the owner, remembers us from our last visit and we chat in French, which always makes me happy. With the bistro vibe and classic French music playing in the background, we briefly imagine ourselves in a little café on the Left Bank. Afterwards we walk down to the foreshore where the stormy weather has piled heaps of seaweed along the beach. We were here in January, on a shimmeringly hot summer's day, and the contrast is stark. But I like the wildness. We then track back to the town for some shopping before heading home in the late afternoon.

I have a quick cycle around the bay for a burst of fresh air before we settle in for the evening. Ian is loving the Tour de France. Today it's the climb up Mont Ventoux, which he proudly conquered in 2018 when he cycled from the north to the south of France, one of his many cycling adventures in Europe that year. He also climbed Tourmalet, another iconic peak from the Tour. That's my man. That's my MAMIL.

I can't really settle and start to pack up for our departure, sorting out clothes and towels and the remaining food in the fridge. We'll take our time tomorrow, make the most of the day and leave in the evening. There's another two weeks until my scan and biopsy. It's been weighing heavily on my mind. I need to find some jobs to do back home, a few projects to keep me busy. I just want to get to this next hurdle and do whatever needs to be done, or hopefully not done, and move on. I want my life back.

13 July 2021
Keep on walking

I don't mind the winter, and we need the rain, but this is getting a bit ridiculous. It's been raining non-stop for the last few days, stormfront after stormfront blowing in across the ocean. On Sunday the downpour was of such biblical proportions that at one point Ian and Ben had to stand in their bathers in our courtyard, as it rapidly turned into a swimming pool, brushing back the water to prevent it from flooding the house. If we hadn't been home the damage would have been substantial. We later saw on the news that many parts of Perth were, indeed, flooded.

I don't know where the time has gone since we came back from Dunsborough. It was nice to see Ben and Ellie and resume normal family life, whatever normal means. My energy and mood vacillate as next week's appointments loom large, despite all my efforts and proclamations about living in the moment.

I finally got to grips with the government website. I'm now proudly vaccinated with my first dose of Pfizer and will have my second dose in three weeks. I didn't feel a thing and had no side-effects apart from a mildly sore arm at the point of entry. Since the standing ovation at Wimbledon, I've read more about the two female scientists who created Astra Zeneca, and their team, and intend to read their book, *Vaxxers*. I'm so sick of misinformation, mixed messages, empty rhetoric and hesitancy. *Come on Australia,* I want to shout from the rooftops, *let's get this done so we can live our lives again.* There's nothing to fear but fear itself.

The array of sport on TV has continued to be a welcome distraction, even though England lost the Euro final on penalties – goddammit! A handsome Italian lost the Wimbledon men's tennis final, but our very own Ash Barty was victorious in the women's final, and a more worthy champion you could never find. Ash Barty for Prime Minister, that's what I say. She's talented, humble, articulate, intelligent, grounded.

I look out the window and can see there's a break in the rain so I might head out for a walk. After my vaccination, I made the most of a two-hour dry spell for a speedy hike around Bold Park before the heavens opened again. Rain or shine, I'm determined to keep on walking.

18 July 2021
The state of the nation

10.25 am
The weekend paper makes for depressing reading. One article comments starkly on the state we're in, on: "… the narcissism of our power-crazed premiers who … talk up threats and assume the role of protector by seizing additional powers … (who) urged on by sensationalist media and encouraged by a public they have deliberately frightened, have convinced themselves that the only metric on their performance is the number of infections." The author's insights about his own profession are chilling: "Instead of

encouraging debate and probing alternatives, most journalists join politicians in trying to scare the public into following instructions and shaming someone for not wearing a mask."

It's powerful stuff and I find myself concurring with much of what he writes about the mayhem and misconceptions that have infected our country more than COVID itself. But then I wonder if he isn't just adding to public fear with the vehemence of his condemnation of the media and our leaders.

Equally chilling is an opinion piece that ended with this damning conclusion: "Hide from the virus. Hide from the world, even as it opens up. This is what our leaders have condemned us to, seemingly in perpetuity. Our situation is beyond parody, and beyond pathetic."

The writer of the first article claims this is not the Australia he knows. Sadly, I tend to agree – this is not the land I emigrated to 20 years ago. Whatever happened to "we are one ... we share a dream and sing with one voice?" I wonder again. Where has the resilience and togetherness gone, the realism and common sense? I'm worried for the future, fearful that that the hardline restrictions and slow vaccination uptake will keep my family splintered for years to come. We can't hide from the world forever.

Later

Yesterday was our wedding anniversary – 28 years. And they told me it wouldn't last! In the early days of our relationship, when Ian and I lived a world apart for over a year, a few naysayers predicted the failure of our union with their "long distance romances never work" pronouncements and unhelpful queries about how we were possibly going to make it happen.

We celebrated quietly. We didn't proclaim the occasion publicly or declare our never-ending love for each other and the perfection of our life together on Facebook. No life is perfect. No marriage is flawless. Ian hid a sweet little card, with a heartfelt message, under the newspaper he often delivers to me after his Saturday morning ride. I made him a photo video of memories, for his eyes only. We went for a long walk in the wind and drizzle, remembering past anniversaries, reminiscing about the times when we were able to spend them in some hidden corner of Europe, in the days when we could travel, remembering our beginnings, the songs we used to listen to, that night in an Essex pub when the penny began to drop … we were always a slow burn.

Later, we watched Ben's hockey match, and in the evening had dinner at a local French restaurant. It was lovely to be out, to chat to the staff, to hear the strains of Edith Piaf as we ate our boeuf bourguignon and cracked the crust on our crème brulées and sipped our wine, a smooth cabernet merlot from the Bordeaux region.

Today, I'm still melancholic about the state of the nation, and apprehensive about my appointments this week, a scan tomorrow and the biopsy on Thursday. That will be the big one, the one I've been doing all I can to forget about until the day arrives. I've done a good job on the whole, of getting on with things, of going about my life as if I didn't have the possibility of another malignancy hanging over me. There'll be yet another two weeks of waiting after the biopsy. I'm hoping that by my birthday, August 4, I'll know the result. I'm wishing for the best present ever, hoping to hear words like *benign*, or *no malignancy*, *nothing to worry about, this part of your body is clear.*

I will be well, I will be well, I will be well. I've got this.

Ian goes back to work tomorrow as the new term commences. Ever conscientious, he's in the office this morning setting up experiments, planning the weeks ahead. By mid-term I hope to be planning my return to work.

In the meantime, I'll keep doing what I've been doing:

Number one: Walking through the wind and rain – the rain is set to continue for some time yet, if the forecast is correct. It won't keep me inside. As the saying goes, "there's no such thing as bad weather, just bad clothes."

Number two: feeling gratitude every day. I don't use that word lightly. I know from experience that gratitude is one of the greatest tools for fighting despair, that building a practice of gratitude creates joy, even in the midst of turmoil and uncertainty. I've come to learn that *#grateful*, or *#gratitude* is far more than some empty platitude attached to a carefully curated Instagram post, but a way of life that reaps endless rewards. I've come to see that gratitude works, by expanding our capacity for the accumulation of joy. By giving us perspective and resilience through good times and bad.

Gratitude doesn't mean we stop feeling pain, but it makes it much more bearable if we never lose sight of joy and wonder. I knew all this before the advent of Alan but had stopped making it a priority. It took Alan for me to see that I was suffering the consequences and experiencing a joy deficit. How ironic that these past four months have helped me work on my practice of gratitude, and experience greater joy (and I'm so grateful for that!).

Number three: doing strength, flexibility and stretching exercises every day, however I'm feeling. It's not negotiable.

Number four: reading, every day. I always have at least one book on the go, in hard copy or Kindle form, or one of each. I read, therefore I think, therefore I write, therefore I am.

Number five: listening to music. I need a daily soundtrack, if only in the background of my life. Sometimes I need music for its own sake, not as an accompaniment to any other activity. Sometimes I need it as much as I need to breathe the air. Music is always there to pull me out of destructive or negative thought patterns.

Number six: Writing this journal, this hotchpotch of thoughts from the mundane to the fanciful and, dare I suggest, the profound, has provided surprising insight into my own life. Whatever it becomes in the future, this regular practice of documenting one of the toughest times I've ever experienced, of using my words to process hard things, is the best form of therapy. I highly recommend writing to anyone doing it tough.

Number seven: listening to podcasts. Current favourites are *Unlocking Us* and *Dare to Lead*, *Armchair Expert* and the new spin-off, *Shattered Glass*; *Chat 10 looks 3* – I've got tickets to see the live Chat 10 show here in Perth in September – please don't let it be cancelled due to lockdowns; *Desert Islands Discs* – it has an amazing back catalogue; *All in the Mind*, a BBC mental health podcast; *In Our Time*, another BBC gem, and many more.

I've continued listening to the *Sister Strong* series on *Unlocking Us*, in which Brené and her sisters review the guideposts outlined in her book *The Gifts of Imperfection*. They tell me I must prioritise myself as much as I can. That if my light is dim, I need people who will allow it to be dim and who will stay by my side, no matter what. That I need to let go of fear and powerlessness. That we have a collective fear of grief, and that grief is not just about death, but about any kind of deep loss.

Another interviewee this week reminded me that we could quite easily fill our days simply responding to other people's expectations of us, and that we need to clear everything off our mental agenda that isn't relevant. That spending time each day clearing our email inboxes is a Sisyphean, and therefore pointless and unproductive, task. That responding and reacting to constant demands is a huge threat to thinking deeply and creatively. Amen to all of that.

I could go on, but I like the number seven, so will stop there.

19 July 2021
Back in the headlights

The day of the CT neck scan is finally here. It's the start of a tough week as all the cancer stuff moves back into the headlights. My equanimity deserts me. I feel edgy and anxious once more.

To distract myself I read Nicki Gemmell's piece on friendship in the *Weekend Australian* magazine while drinking my coffee. What she writes mirrors exactly the way I feel: "Real friendship is about being vulnerable with each other in terms of the complexities of our lives … honesty connects … I don't want to waste precious time on those who exhaust me, nibble away at my equilibrium, flatten with little barbs. If I don't feel like someone's got my back, honestly, what's the point?"

I couldn't agree more. All too often I allow people to nibble away at my equilibrium. But I'm getting better at being more discerning when it comes to sifting out those who, as Nikki laments, "rattle rather than nourish the soul". We all need to avoid the "heart-sinkers" and seek out the "heart-lifters" because life is too short to spend with "those who make us lesser".

I drive to the radiology clinic for the scan. All runs smoothly, but as I present my arm for the canula to be inserted so the contrast can be administered through my veins I'm suddenly overcome with emotion. Tears well up. I want to howl, *not again, please god, not again*. The radiologist keeps asking if I'm OK. I can't speak, but I nod and give her a half-hearted thumbs up. I'm not afraid of the needle or the canula or the machine. I'm not claustrophobic. But I hate all this. I've had weeks of freedom, of semi-normality, and now I'm back on the medical treadmill and I want to get off.

My agitation continues throughout the day. I keep telling myself to breathe and let the feelings be what they are, but it's hard. Ian is going to see his parents this afternoon as it's Pam's birthday tomorrow, so after the scan I go present shopping but can't find her favourite perfume anywhere. I end up buying a book and some fancy nougat before rushing home to drive Ian to the station in between appointments – I have yet another one later today with a dermatologist. Ian is taking the train instead of driving to his parents's place so he can get some work done on the journey. I'm grumpy in the car, drained by all that is happening and silently regretting my offer to help Ian out with the present buying and lift to the station. I shouldn't be resentful, I know, and feel like a complete shit for feeling as I do. Useless and worthless. A terrible person.

I try to calm down at home, eat lunch and chill out with John Mayer, who never fails to lift my mood. At the dermatology appointment we discuss trying a new drug to better control the eczema that has been a constant since birth and has been particularly bad of late. I'm keen to see if anything can be done to improve my skin and reduce flare-ups. We start the ball rolling today, but it will be a while before anything happens. I have other fish to fry. But it's a start, at least.

I keep working on my mood as the day continues and manage to maintain some degree of control. Awareness is the key. Awareness of the shittiness of my mood and the willingness to let it be as shitty as it needs to be until it works itself through. The house is quiet, which is just what I need. Ian won't be back until later and Ben is out. I make a quick meal and escape into the last two episodes of *Belgravia* on iView. When Ian and Ben return, we don't talk much, but there's no acrimony. Just a tacit acknowledgement that I've struggled today. There's always tomorrow. Maybe the sun will come out (fat chance).

20 July 2021
Hoping for a miracle

I have a meeting at the Curriculum Authority this morning, which takes my mind off things. The project is almost complete. The discussions are productive and affirming; I'm pleased with my leadership and the team effort.

I take my time getting home and am just about to stop off for some food shopping when Tony calls about the CT scan.

'There's no real change,' he tells me, and my heart sinks.

I was secretly hoping for a miracle, hoping the scan would be clear and a further biopsy unnecessary, but no such miracle occurs.

It hits me hard when he hangs up. I need to focus on the road but I'm suddenly very scared as reality looms large, the reality that something nasty may be revealed and that I may need further treatment. I know I'll somehow find the strength to deal with the worst-case scenario should it occur but feel physically sick at the thought.

21 July 2021
The comfort of toast

I wake in turmoil after tortured dreams with a growing sense of panic about tomorrow. Then I make myself a late breakfast and wonder if there's anything better in the world than butter and marmalade liberally spread on toast made from home-baked sourdough, washed down with a steaming mug of proper strong Yorkshire tea. I decide that in this emotional rollercoaster world of mine there isn't. Anything better, that is.

1.30 pm
Listen

Georgia calls as we arranged a few days ago. It's 6.30 am in England, but she's an early riser and the timing suits us both. She's just back from a week in Cornwall, is enjoying her new job and feeling more settled in her flat. I tell her about my angst and fear of what tomorrow may bring.

She listens without interruption. How many people do that, listen until you've finished what you need to say, without interjecting for the sake of it? It's rare and refreshing. So many people interrupt before you've had a chance to express what you want to say, jumping in with their take on things before they even know what the things really are, or reciting some unhelpful experience of their own.

We talk for an hour or so before Georgia starts work. She's still working from home. I'm interested to find out how she stays motivated and disciplined. She tells me there's a clear structure to each day and she has no problem staying on task. The plan is for employees to eventually spend three days every fortnight in the office, but otherwise continue to work remotely. It sounds ideal. Change to the way we work is one of the positives to come out of COVID.

I don't want to talk about medical details, but I tell Georgia I'm shit scared about tomorrow. I'm not looking for answers. I don't expect her to fix me. I just need to speak my thoughts out loud, and it's so helpful, such a relief and release to talk when you know you're being heard, when there's a soft place where your feelings can land.

22 July 2021
Gratitude and joy

Tomorrow is here. The scary thing is happening. I'm in hospital again, on a bed in the day ward, gown on, endless forms filled in, waiting, just waiting. The 6.30 am start was as brutal as the artificial lights in the admissions reception area. In my sleep-deprived, anxiety-ridden state, I close my eyes against the harsh brightness, trying to calm my mind. I want all of this to be over. I want it all to go away.

Six hours later I'm back home, feeling OK apart from some mild to moderate pain and a scratchy throat. The fear has all but gone. It's done. I didn't die on the operating table. Maybe because it's been such a long wait to get to this day, I'd created some crazy scenarios in my head about the procedure itself as much as the outcome, imagined all the things that could go wrong after reading through the potential risks when I signed the authority to proceed with surgery. Best not to read and just sign, perhaps.

Tony calls to see how I am and apologises for not seeing me before I left hospital. He'll see me next week for the histology report. Another scary thing that I must try to "park", as he told me months ago, somewhere far out of reach for the time being. I have no control over the results. They will be what they already are.

I need to go and get me some joy. With that intent, I step outside and look through the trees and across rooftops towards the horizon.

And there it is; the light. There's a certain time each afternoon when the stretch of ocean visible in the distance from the back of our house transforms into a sheet of shimmering silvery light. How wonderful it would be, I often think, to bathe in that liquid light, to lose myself in its iridescence, to let it infuse my body and mind, to make me shiny and new with its healing power, to soothe my soul and replenish my spirit.

As I stare in awe, I give thanks for this day, for Tony's surgical expertise, for Deepak the anaesthetist, for the nurses and porters and for the hospital itself for being a place where I could, once more, be investigated and cared for.

It was a different hospital from last time, but everything was so familiar: the bright lights, the sexy gown and cap, the smiling staff, my shivering on the operating table in the cold, cold theatre, the warm blankets, Tony and Deepak smiling and reassuring in their scrubs.

'It's really good to see you,' said Tony. 'We'll get this all sorted out.'

Then the sharp prick in my arm before the sink into oblivion, the waking up in slight confusion, the hot tea and sandwiches.

It's done now, I think again, and with the gratitude comes a sudden surge of joy as I gaze towards the light. Joy is possible, even on this difficult day, even at this time of uncertainty, even as I must wait yet again to find out my fate. I hold the joy tight and tie it up with a ribbon in my mind.

24 July 2021
Recovery

I'm not doing very much except resting and recovering. My throat is sore, I've had some nausea and feel more tired than usual, all quite normal post-surgery reactions. I'm eating well and have been out for short walks. Last night I cooked a delicious chilli con carne for dinner and today I've made a huge pot of chicken soup to see us through the next few days. I'm caring for myself and feeding my family. It feels nice.

Ben is in and out of the house, out more often than in, and we haven't talked much lately about what's going on in my life. I think he still finds it a bit confronting and doesn't quite know what to say or how he should react. I want to chat about how he's dealing with everything and reassure him that there's no "should", but before I can he's off again, called suddenly into work. That's Ben. Always busy, always on the go. It sometimes feels as though he's slipping through my fingers, moving away, untangling himself from my apron strings.

The garden project is advancing slowly. We're making appointments to get quotes from a few landscapers. Ian and Ben have been pulling out old plants and weeds. I even had a go myself and was surprised at the small pleasure of hands in soil. The garden looks like a blank canvas waiting to be brought to life. It's exciting, something to look forward to. I want to be part of the creative process as we develop an outdoor space worthy of the house we so lovingly renovated. I want my own little slice of Eden, a haven to feed the soul and carry me through whatever lies ahead.

25 July 2021
Panic and despair

I can't find the joy today and don't want to get out of bed. I've slept for hours but don't have the energy to do anything. I can barely drag myself to the kitchen to make a cup of tea. This rollercoaster is relentless. I'm up, then down, then down some more, then up a bit before the steepest descent into panic and despair. I find myself wishing for the rollercoaster to malfunction, for a technical error to send my car off the rails, plummeting to the ground below, crashing into blessed oblivion.

26 July 2021
Olympic dreams

The panic continues and I start the week with an all-consuming sense of dread. *I Don't Like Mondays* was a classic anthem of my youth. I don't much like any day at the moment. This waiting is excruciating. I can't pull myself out of the funk of fear I've fallen into, all because of a shadow on a scan that has been inconclusively investigated for months.

I hope last week's biopsy will finally give me an answer. I couldn't bear any more inconclusivity (is that a word?). I need to know so I can deal with whatever has to be done. I tell Ian I don't think I can cope with any more treatment. If the news is not good on Friday I'd prefer to be put out of my misery.

'What happened to "I've got this"?' he asks me gently. 'You've come through before and you will again. I'm here. Stay strong. We'll face it together.'

'I don't feel strong,' I tell him. 'I feel beaten down by fear. That was then and this is now.'

Thank god for the Olympics. The Australian swimming team is on fire. It's uplifting and inspirational to watch, even in my agitated state. It's joyous, in fact. It keeps on surprising me that I can still experience joy amidst the angst. I cling to that as I urge the swimmers on, sitting up in bed watching the finals in my pyjamas, cheering at every gold and silver and bronze medal, delighting in the back stories, the triumph over adversity, the years of toil and sweat that led to this moment and the tears that flow post-performance in victory or disappointment. And then there's the swimmer whose father died from brain cancer a year ago, who's competing in his memory. Cancer. It's everywhere.

In the afternoon a landscaper comes to look at our garden. He has some good ideas and seems to understand my garbled explanation of what we're looking for. We'll see if his quote correlates in any way with our meagre budget. I hope so. I want to watch things grow and flourish and fruit and blossom.

27 July 2021
RIP old friend

I'm hanging by a thread as Friday approaches, the day when I'll find out whether I need more treatment, whether Alan has an equally evil twin. I now know what it means to be worried sick. My mother used that expression a lot. Worrying was part of her DNA.

Like mother, like daughter. I've been sick in my stomach for days now, sick with worry about what will happen. Nauseous and emotionally drained and anxious in a way I can't seem to shake. My anxiety levels are off the scale.

I hit yet another low point when I find out on Facebook that a colleague and friend from our County Durham days has died. As well as being an inspirational music teacher, musician, organist and choir master, Paul was an amazing human: kind, generous, curious and full of zest for living. He was a wonderful cook and loved to host dinner parties for his many friends from the school and the broader town community. Paul played the organ at Daniel's christening in the school chapel. I sang in the choir he conducted, performed Handel's *Messiah* at Christmas in the town hall to the rhythm of his expert baton. We saw him almost every day for four years, shared so much of our lives, including a holiday in Cornwall when I was pregnant with Daniel. Life was endless fun when Paul was around.

Sadly, we lost touch over the years, but I had some sporadic contact with him on Facebook in the last couple of years.

I don't know any details except that he had finally hung up his teaching baton last year and been in hospital for two weeks prior to his death. It seems beyond cruel that he didn't get a chance to enjoy his retirement. I tell Ian the shocking news when he gets home; he can't believe it. Why do good people die before their time?

I message some mutual friends in sadness and disbelief and arrange to chat with Marion tomorrow. We've been meaning to catch up for some time and after yesterday's news I want to talk about Paul and remember him with someone who knew him too. And I want to hear her voice and hear all her news. We haven't seen or spoken to each other since 2016.

Why do people I know, people around my age, keep dying? I don't usually mind being on my own but I'm finding it unbearable now. I cry on and off all day thinking of Paul and sickness and death and want to scream at the unfairness of it all.

Sydney is in lockdown again, so I call Anne to find out how they're coping. Her daughter is in Year 12, which isn't easy during a pandemic. There's a lot of uncertainty about whether the HSC exams will go ahead. So much is on hold. So many lives are impacted. Will it ever end?

28 July 2021
So far apart

The Olympics continue, providing entertainment and inspiration all morning, taking my mind off biopsies and scans and all the horrible medical stuff. One of the Australian swimmers was in my French class many years ago, and Ben plays club hockey with one of the Kookaburras, the Australian men's hockey team, which makes it even more exciting to watch their performances.

Right on the dot of 4.00 pm, the time we had arranged, Marion and I call each other simultaneously. It feels like five minutes rather than five years since we were together. Steve is with her, making his characteristic wisecracks and oh my goodness, I love these people. The connection is strong, the understanding is mutual, the humour is still there, the friendship is unbreakable. We catch up on all the news from our lives and laugh and cry and say we should do this more often and make tentative plans for future holidays and it feels so lovely and right and warm and why, oh why, do we have to live so far apart?

29 July 2021
Paralysis

I can't muster the energy to get out of bed today, so I stay put until Ian comes home from school. I'm paralysed with fear and take refuge in the Olympics again, and whatever else is on TV, trying to numb myself with the screen. He cuddles me and tells me to come out into the garden so I can tell him which branches to chop down from the tree in the middle. I tell him I don't smell so good and need to shower and get dressed before heading out into the garden.

It's blowing a gale, so he doesn't chop the branches, but I'm grateful he got me out of bed. I relish the wind in my face and take the dog for a walk instead.

I tell Ian I don't know if I can do this alone tomorrow, I don't know if I can drive to the clinic to get my results and I don't know what I'll do if the news is not good. So we plan for either Ian or Ben to drive me there and pick me up.

30 July 2021
Walking in a straight line

Something shifts in the night. I get up feeling stronger and make my own way to the ENT clinic to find out my fate. I'm expecting the worst. I park some distance away so I can walk for 20 minutes to get to the clinic. Through my headphones Daniel Johns sings about walking in a straight line, and I vow to do just that. I see lots of little furry caterpillars on the paths as I walk and wonder if they are very hungry.

For once the appointments are running on time and I'm ushered straight into the consulting room. After a few minutes Tony breezes in and tells me it's all good. I don't quite know what to say. "All good" was not what I was expecting to hear.

'The nodule is benign,' he continues. 'And the lymph node has reduced in size since your first scan, so it's no longer a cause for concern.'

He qualifies all of this with more explanation about nothing ever being 100 percent and wanting to monitor things and telling me he'd like to see me again in six months but that I'm not going to die of tongue or throat or neck cancer anytime soon. He tells me all of this in a strange kind of deadpan way (maybe he's had a tough morning in theatre), which I comment on, wanting a little more reassurance or emotion, or something. He then tells me he's very happy for me and that I'll come out of all this a stronger person and that I must now go and enjoy my life.

It's all a bit odd, and something of an anticlimax, despite being the hugest (who cares if that's not a word) relief ever. Afterwards I realise, with no small amount of shame, that this kind of conversation is all in a day's work for Tony, that he may well have to tell other people less good news, that doing the job he does must require some reining in of emotion, that the world does not revolve around me.

Tony's receptionist shares my relief and hugs me long and hard when I come out of the consultation. I put my head down on her desk and just breathe for a while, letting it all sink in, the sweet relief.

All that fucking worry for nothing. That'll teach me. Or will it? If it doesn't, it damn well should.

I message Ian and Ben with the news and walk back to the car the long way round through Kings Park. When I emerge from the bush into an open space, I notice something I hadn't seen before; a stone labyrinth. As a child I loved Greek mythology and was fascinated by the story of Ariadne's glittering thread. I walk slowly through the maze of paths, hitting every dead end until I make it to the centre where I stand for a while in contemplation before taking the quickest route out. Like Theseus, I have slain the Minotaur and found my way out of the maze.

I stop off at a supermarket and fill my basket with serrano ham and stuffed Spanish olives and squishy cheese and gourmet pâté and high-quality bacon and freshly squeezed juice and Simmo's ice-cream. The woman at the checkout does that thing good salespeople do to make you feel pleased about your purchases, commenting on each item, saying either how delicious it is, what a good choice I've made, or what a great price it is. And it works. I feel very good indeed about my purchases and pretty damn great about the rest of this precious day as I drive home knowing that Alan does not have an evil twin in my body.

As for Alan himself, well, a couple of months ago I was told it looked as though he was no more. I didn't quite believe it, and I won't fully believe it until the next check in September. But for now, I owe it to myself, and to all those who have walked with me through this unexpected chapter of my life, to enjoy each and every day and make the most of what I have.

There is still much mind work to be done. This, I know. I beat depression years ago, but anxiety still circles around and all too often stops me from living my best life. I will attend to that in due course.

For now, though, it's enough to be here. I think of my friends and all the conversations that have sustained me. They have lifted me up more than they will ever know.

I message Anne, Steve and Marion, a French friend, and more. I message Georgia on WhatsApp and ask if she's free to chat. I fill her in on the non-existence of Alan's evil twin, about whom she had no idea, and all the anxiety that imaginary entity has caused me.

'I didn't tell anyone,' I say to her. 'Except for Ian and Ben, because it was all too confronting to have to talk about another potential malignancy and the possibility of more treatment being needed. I just didn't want to, couldn't bear to, share that.'

'I wanted to tell you in person, to hear your voice,' I continue, and then I just break down, in the best possible way, as all the pent-up emotion overflows. Georgia needs to get to work but we'll talk again very soon.

Marita next. It's been a while, too long. I tell her my news and we debrief on the last couple of months. For the first time, I tell her about naming my cancer Alan, and she loves it, and we laugh and laugh and laugh some more. She asks about my writing and I tell her I've nearly written another book. This book. That after today I can write the ending. Or some sense of an ending. For this story is not completely over, as anyone who has ever had cancer will know. There will be scans and checks for years to come.

Five years ago, I sat in a corner of Marita's apartment in Melbourne, laptop on my knee, lost in the world of words, writing the last chapter and epilogue of my first book. I was barely aware of her as I wrote, but felt the subconscious comfort of her presence as she sorted out her wardrobe for the working week ahead, and planned and prepped and chopped and cooked, and put yummy things into containers and freezer bags, and labelled them all with her immaculate calligraphy, and stored them systematically for the coming weeks. I sensed the contentment of her creating and organising as I wrote.

Occasionally, I would briefly glance at her or stare through the window across the rooftops of South Yarra as a fresh thought or new sentence formed in my head. It was the most comfortable of silences. Two old friends just doing their thing.

When I finally emerged from that blessed state of flow and looked up for more than a few seconds, Marita was staring at me as if in awe. I had no idea that several hours had passed.

'I always knew you loved to write, Suze,' she said. 'But now I see, now I know you really are a writer.'

Marita was the first person to read my manuscript and give me feedback, the first person who really believed in my writing and encouraged my dream of becoming an author.

'Why am I not surprised you've written another book,' she says now, across the country from Melbourne to Perth. 'You're a writer, my friend. That's what you are and that's what you must continue to do.'

1 August 2021
One of the lucky ones

I will be 59 in three days. The early birthday present I'd hoped for is slowly sinking in – the gift of good news. I know I'll be back and forward for scans and checks for years to come, but I need to savour the here and now and rejoice in the knowledge that there's no secondary cancer and that my treatment seems to have succeeded in killing Alan. It's a lot to process. That's why I keep saying "seem". There are further hoops to jump through before I'm satisfied that Alan is well and truly dead.

I started celebrating my birth week yesterday with a glass of champagne at lunch with a friend. As we sat overlooking the ocean we both love, she filled me in on her husband's cancer battle. When COVID changed the world, the drug he was trialing, and to which he had been responding well, was withdrawn. He's now on immunotherapy, responding positively and doing the best he can, but they're acutely aware their time is limited.

We all have limited time; our days on this earth are not infinite. As I sat with my friend and we talked, with the ocean roaring below us, I was profoundly aware, and deeply grateful, that I am one of the lucky ones.

'How lucky we are to be here now,' she commented, as if reading my thoughts. My friend's strength is immense. Her spirit fills the room. Her light shines brightly. Her essence is pure and good. The world needs more people like this friend of mine.

When I get home, I message Lorna with my news and she replies straight away with an ecstatic 'Call me!' I tell her about the non-existence of the evil twin and my growing confidence about Alan's demise. She's overjoyed. Our conversation fills me to the brim. We have an innate understanding of each other, a connection that began back in the 1980s when we wore big earrings and even bigger hair and ridiculous shoulder pads and thick black eyeliner and thought we were absolutely fabulous. I love this girl to the moon and back. She opens up something ancient and primal inside me, something precious and eternal.

I'm slowly gaining a sense of the enormity of all of this, of Alan and his potential evil twin and of their demise. They say that cancer changes people. That you're never the same again. I think that must be true of any trauma or major illness. They create new layers within you, reveal hidden depths, offer different perspectives; layers and depths and perspectives that make up a person and form a lifetime of human experience on this tiny planet spinning within a vast and mysterious universe.

6 August 2021

Happy birthday to me!

I've been out to lunch and dinner twice in the last week. That's more socialising than I've done in a long time. I'm tired now and need time out to rest over the weekend before heading south again on Monday, back to the sanctuary of Geographe Bay where I will finish and edit this book before sending it to my writer friend. My words need fresh eyes now. I'm apprehensive, but mostly excited, that she'll be reading my work and that I'll have the chance to learn more about writing from a professional. We had a birthday-eve dinner on Tuesday night to discuss the book, among many other things: COVID, our second vaccines booked coincidentally at the same place at more or less the same time this week, politicians, family, work life balance, retirement, superannuation and everything in between. I'm always energised by her company.

Ben and his friend Emily, who has been a great source of comfort and distraction for him through all of this, took me out for a birthday lunch at a French restaurant. Food that never disappoints, and attentive service, has made it a family favourite for special occasions. Today is no exception. Ben and Emily provide sparkling company and Ben picks up the bill. I'm not losing him. He's not slipping through my fingers. He's just growing up.

To end the birthday week, Ian and I had dinner with friends in a quirky little bar that serves great share plates, always a fun way to eat. The bar was Friday-night packed, but we struck lucky with a waitress who attended to our every need with grace and humour, despite the pressure of a busy night's service. We enjoyed a wonderful evening eating delicious food and drinking fine wine with good friends.

When I suggested a generous tip, Ian looked at me in amazement, made some quip about the rarity of my suggestion, and laughed at his own hilarity. I do indeed rarely tip but am more than happy to dig deep when the service warrants acknowledgement, and on that night it did.

Life is good and all is well.

7 August 2021
Days like these reprise

It's been four and a half months since my GP took one look at my backside and picked up the phone, 136 days since my world was turned upside down and back to front.

I sit staring through the window to the horizon on another stormy Saturday, thinking about days like these.

On days like these I hear that my cancer has responded well to treatment and my tumour appears to be no more. On days like these I am filled with the relief and release of finding out I do not, after all, have a secondary cancer as I drive to have lunch with a friend and discuss exciting new possibilities.

On days like these I bump into Nurse Jacky, my finger saviour, at the beach and tell her my news and we hug and I shed a tear as we walk together along the water's edge and chat and laugh and marvel at how lucky we are to have this beautiful beach and endless ocean on our doorstep, particularly during a global pandemic.

On days like these I am not afraid of anything and everything seems possible.

On days like these I am unencumbered by emotional baggage.

On days like these I can forgive, forget and let it all go.

On days like these I wish nothing but love and light to my fellow humans.

On days like these my serenity knows no bounds.

On days like these I give thanks for the gift of life.

9 August 2021
Family matters 2

I'm driving south again for another mini-retreat while I still can, reflecting on all that has happened in the last week as I listen to a playlist of eighties hits.

Before leaving, I went to school to change my password and install some updates. It seemed like a good opportunity to attend Monday morning briefing, show my face again and start discussing time-tabling options for Term 4. It was nice to be back, or at least to be on the way back. My request to return on a part-time basis has been verbally acknowledged and approved so I can look forward to a lighter load when I return.

I finally emailed my brother and sister to tell them what's been going on in my life. My brother sent a card for my birthday, so I used that as an opener, and I'd yet to reply to the email my sister sent after her birthday last month.

Credit and deep thanks must go to my five-year old great-niece (and her mum) for giving me the courage and push I needed to get in touch when they sent an adorable video message about my picture books. *Pink*, the first one I wrote, is dedicated to her.

'Hello Great Aunty Sue (I know, I'm a dinosaur),' she said on the video. 'I love this book and read it all the time. I can't wait to read all the rest. Thanks for writing them.'

I messaged straight back to tell her how pleased I was, thanked her for sending such a lovely message and encouraged her to keep reading.

It was one of those online exchanges that gather momentum and flow effortlessly. My niece is going to buy the rest of the books and wanted to know the best way to do that (I could send them, but Amazon is probably quicker, given the current state of the postal service). I congratulated her on a new job as deputy principal and she shared some more news before I took a deep breath and told her about being diagnosed with cancer back in March.

'You're the first person in the family to know,' I said.

'Does that include Dad (my brother)?' she asked.

'Yes, and my sister. I just haven't felt able to tell them. It's all been so confronting.'

We continued messaging for a while about this, that and the other, and family matters, and when we signed off I'd more or less decided the time was right to get in touch.

I almost broke down when I received prompt replies to the emails I sent the next day to my brother and sister. They both expressed their sorrow and sent their love and support and concern for all of us. I couldn't have asked for more heartwarming messages. I think we all know our relationships are complicated, that our family, like many others, has its own dysfunctions and past traumas that can sometimes be hard to navigate. But there's always love, of that I'm sure. We just need to become better at expressing it.

For some reason, my illness brought up a lot of family baggage and I wasn't ready to share such difficult and personal news until now. But I'm so glad I did.

I also posted a blog on my website called *Fighting Cancer in the Time of COVID*. I figured it was time to feel the fear and share it anyway. The response I received from friends around the world, the outpouring of love, support and kindness was overwhelming and humbling. People contacted me to share their own cancer experiences, I found out that a friend has just lost her mother, that another is still recovering from a bitter separation, and yet another is now thriving after being through both depression and cancer, just like me.

Everyone is going through something. We all have a story to tell. This is life, and life is messy and glorious and sad and joyful all at the same time. People get sick, some recover and some don't. Death is part of life and we need to talk about it more.

Months ago, I wondered what kind of a cancer patient I would be. I think the answer is that I was my own kind of patient. You can only be who and how you are. There is no right or wrong way to be. I've been sad, happy, grumpy, patient, irritable, accepting, selfish, kind, despairing, joyful. I'm a mass of contradictions, a perfectly imperfect human recovering from an illness that affects one in two people at some time in their lives.

When I look back at what I wrote as I slowly emerged from the fog of depression, I find so much that resonates with my battle with cancer. I came to see that depression and anxiety did not need to be a life sentence and was determined they would not define me. I learned that with patience, persistence and determination you can find your way out of the darkness and live a life that's fuller, more joyful and more meaningful than before.

Through my two health crises I have learned just how much I love and am loved. I have learned to cherish the amazing friends I have the world over.

I have learned that we need to follow our passions and seek out the things we enjoy and that make our hearts sing. That we all have the power to create inside of us; we just need to dig deep sometimes in order to find our creative talents. That in exploring our spiritual side we move beyond ourselves and our egos.

I have learned that while grief and suffering and loss shape our lives, they neither define us nor prevent us from experiencing great joy. I have learned that if I am not there for myself I cannot possibly be there for everyone else, and I have learned that I cannot be all things to all people at any given time.

I have learned that laughter is excellent medicine and that the best comedy is often born out of misfortune, that humour helps us to survive and deal with our own inadequacies. I have learned that there are lots of things I still want to do in my remaining time on this earth.

Fighting cancer can feel like a very lonely battle, a gruelling, spirit-sapping duel, a mind-draining waiting game that seems as if it will never end. But I know that I am one of millions, that I am not alone. I also know that the best thing I can do now, for my own sake and for the sake of all those I love and who love me, is to make the most of the gift of life. And just keep walking.

Encore

I'm sitting on the beach under a canopy of soft blue sky dotted with pink-tinged clouds, gazing at the gentle winter colour palette mirrored in the rippling waters of Geographe Bay. It's been stormy for days but this evening all is calm, with just a hint of a breeze. The tide is slowly creeping in, gradually covering the exposed sand bars and rocks. A lone pelican floats along the horizon, aglow in the rays of the setting sun. Dog walkers chat and throw balls.

I suddenly become aware of a distinct and achingly familiar accent and can't help myself:

'You're from Northern Ireland,' I say to a young father with his family.

'I am indeed,' he replies. 'Where are you from?'

We talk about our homeland for a while, share our immigration stories, reminisce a little, lament the state of the planet and the pain of separation, but agree that we're lucky to be here in this magical place where his children can run free and pick up shells and paddle in safe, shallow water, and find crabs in rockpools and run around barefoot for most of the year.

As darkness descends and people make their way home, I sit on a log and stare across the bay, breathing in the beauty, the wildness, the magic and mystery. The colours darken and sea and sky become one. A crescent moon hangs above a single bright star.

It's some time before I'm aware that silent tears are streaming down my face.

When I was a little girl, a shy, sensitive emotional little girl, I was always told not to cry, told by my parents, teachers and almost everyone I met to suppress my tears when I was upset. The only person who ever acknowledged that it was OK to feel sad was a hockey coach who sat with me when I was sobbing at the front of the school bus on the way to a match one Saturday morning. As the youngest player in the team, who had just displaced an older player, I'd been on the receiving end of some unkind comments from my new teammates, was struggling to fit in and felt unworthy of my place in the squad.

As I sobbed, I remember apologising to my coach for crying, feeling ashamed and embarrassed and telling her it was nothing. She told me that if something had made me this unhappy it was not nothing. My hockey coach was the only adult in my childhood and adolescence who gave me the courage to elaborate on the reason for my tears without admonishing me for shedding them. She sat beside me until my sobbing abated, reassuring me that I had more than earned my spot in the team.

That's the only time I remember an adult affirming my adolescent feelings. I slowly regained confidence on the hockey field, my teammates saw that I was a worthy addition to the squad, and we went on to have the most successful season in years, bringing home the Northern Irish school's trophy. It was one of the happiest times of my school life.

I grew up believing there was something wrong with me because I cried easily and battled so many conflicting emotions. I never felt like I fitted in anywhere and was constantly reminded to rein myself in whenever I tried to express what was inside. Don't be sad but don't be too happy. Don't celebrate when you score a goal, just walk back modestly to the centre line. Don't think about yourself, think about others. Don't be this, don't be that. In other words, don't be who you are, suppress your natural instincts. Obey. Behave. Don't rock the boat.

I didn't know why I seemed so out of step with everyone, why I always felt like an outsider or why I experienced such intense emotion. I didn't know what I needed and wanted. Had I known how to, or dared ask for what I needed and wanted, it would have been framed as selfishness. I was regularly told I was ungrateful and that I mustn't upset my mother, but I never really knew why.

When I found out I had cancer, I cried in disbelief. I sobbed as my GP's receptionist consoled me. I howled and raged when I got home. I wept at the sadness and cruelty of life and screamed in fear, fear that I wasn't ready for this, fear because I didn't want to have to fight for my life, fear because I wasn't ready to die.

Our emotions are just that, ours, and we suppress them at our peril. We need to feel them, acknowledge them, sit with them, work through them and then, and only then, begin to move on.

Over the last few months, I've experienced many different emotions, both positive and negative, difficult and comforting: shock, fear, disbelief, despair, hopelessness, denial, anxiety, anger, loss, resentment, indignation, frustration, mistrust, impatience, vulnerability, acceptance, courage, extreme joy, awe, wonder, gratitude, happiness, relief, trust, contentment, fulfilment, satisfaction, tranquility, love, peace, empathy, equanimity and a renewed appreciation of beauty and nature.

I've felt all of these (and more, no doubt) fully and deeply. I've worked through the tough stuff and rejoiced in the good stuff. My emotions make me human. Understanding and accepting them helps me understand myself, get through hard times and face what may seem like insurmountable challenges. This is me. I don't want to rein in any part of myself.

Take the reins off and let me run freely. Untether me. Don't tell me to shut up and move on, or keep calm and carry on, or pull myself together, or any other of those useless, dangerous, careless maxims uttered in ignorance. Spoken in fear of intense emotion. Only by expressing and facing our emotions can we learn, grow and become better at managing them.

I once wrote that if I could get through depression, I could get through anything. It was a bold claim, but one that has held good so far. Seven years ago, finally owning my emotions allowed me to work my way not just through, but far beyond that depression. Now, in a way I don't really understand, I know I needed a reminder of the lessons I learnt back then, that I needed to rediscover myself yet again. While cancer is brutal and scary and exhausting, in some unfathomable way it has been a gift, an opportunity, to recalibrate and reset.

I have no doubt the lessons I learnt back then helped me face and accept what happened to my body this year and emerge six months later filled with hope and possibilities, knowing that in spite of trauma and pain and suffering and sickness and pandemics, I will never lose sight of wonder and joy.

I also have no doubt that life will continue to throw me curveballs. I plan to hit them all out of the park.

There's joy not far from here, I know there is,
This isn't everything you are
~ Snow Patrol

Bits and Pieces

Whatever gets you through the day

We all have our own way of coping with tough situations. This is most certainly not a self-help book, but I thought it might be useful to share some of the things that sustained my soul, or just helped me lose myself for an hour or two on a particularly crappy day.

Music

I couldn't live without music. It moves me to tears, lifts me up and speaks to something deep within. Spotify is my platform of choice, although I still have a huge stash of CDs and a small collection of vinyl which occasionally gets dusted off for a whirl on the turntable. I have numerous playlists, and while the Spotify tailor-made library is endless, I love to create my own. Here are some of my most listened to artists and playlists this year:

John Mayer – I just love his music. He keeps me company through the highs and lows of life.

Snow Patrol – Saw them in Perth in 2012 and have loved them ever since. Gary Lightbody's voice gets me every time.

R.E.M. – Hearing what I call the "sorry" song stopped me in my tracks in 1984 and I've been revisiting their back catalogue this year.

Gentle Yoga & Stretching – Relaxed vibes for times when I want to bring the tempo down. Everything from Coldplay to Elbow to Adele to Billie Eilish.

Chill – Similar to the above but sprinkled with the likes of Elgar, Wagner, Bach, Pachelbel, Gluck, Barber, Ennio Morricone and even (eek) a bit of Genesis.

Walking back to happiness – Speaks for itself. Uptempo beats that match my stride.

Binaural Beats Meditation – Apparently, this eases me into a theta brainwave state. It certainly helps me to relax.

Taylor Swift (*Evermore* and *Folklore*) – I love the vibe of these two albums and am a big fan of her music in general.

Leeds 80s – Nostalgia times a gazillion. The soundtrack of my misspent student days.

Brit Pop – Back to the 1990s. Oasis, Blur, The Stone Roses, The Charlatans, Manic Street Preachers, Sting (not sure if he classifies as Brit Pop but I love him, despite his tantric pretensions), et al.

Musical theatre – I'm a huge fan and have many soundtracks and selections from the Broadway and West End greats amongst my playlists.

Cathartic Cathedral Choral – There's something about sacred choral music that speaks to my soul, even though I'm in no way a religious person.

Music gives a soul to the universe, wings to the mind, flight to the imagination, and life to everything. ~ Plato

Music, once admitted to the soul, becomes a sort of spirit and never dies. ~ Edward Bulwer-Lytton

Podcasts

I may be technologically challenged but all praise must go to the digital gods for bringing us podcasts. Here are a few favourites that kept me company in hospitals and waiting rooms and helped me get out of my own head:

Chat 10 Looks 3 – (Annabel) Crabb and (Leigh) Sales; say no more. Two leading Australian broadcasters share random musings on books, TV, films, podcasts and life in general. Always a pick-me-up.

Table Manners with Jessie Ware – A delightful series based around food, family and good conversation. Upbeat and life-affirming.

We write the songs with Gary Barlow – The world's leading songwriters share their secrets.

Desert Island Discs – The iconic BBC series with a huge back catalogue to choose from.

All in the Mind – The always thought-provoking BBC mental health programme.

A Bit of Optimism with Simon Sinek – My pick is the episode with comedian Michael McIntyre.

Armchair Expert with Dax Shepard – A celebration of the messiness of being human.

Bryden & – Rob Bryden chats to his friends. Gentle and insightful.

Life's a Beach with Alan Carr – celebrities share their travel tales and favourite destinations.

Unlocking Us with Brené Brown – Lots of inspiration to be found here.

Conversations – Something for everyone on this iconic Radio National series.

In our time: Philosophy – Highbrow conversation courtesy of BBC Radio Four

> *Conversation should touch everything, but should concentrate itself on nothing.* ~ Oscar Wilde

TV

So much choice, so little time. Here is a snippet of what I watched to help me forget about Alan, if only for a while:

The Crown – May not be wholly accurate but I'm a huge fan of this tour de force.

Belgravia – This adaptation of the Julian Fellowes book did not disappoint.

The Capture – A tense ride with the charismatic Callum Turner.

Smother – Power, money, greed and family intrigue on the wild west Irish coast

Innocent – Had to binge it all after the first episode.

Lupin – One of my favourite French actors, Omar Sy, mesmorises in this escapist French adventure series. Stunningly filmed in Paris.

Call my Agent – The fabulous French series that became a global phenomenon.

Little Fires Everywhere – All hail to Reece Witherspoon. An excellent adaptation of the book.

The Queen's Gambit – I don't know anyone who didn't love this.

The Undoing – A standout performance from Hugh Grant. Nicole Kidman not too shabby either.

Unforgotten – Just love the Nicola Walker and Sanjeev Baskar duo and clever plotlines.

Unforgiven – Suranne Jones at her best.

Modern Love – An absolute delight. Loved every minute and cried a lot!

The One – Loved this salutary tale of power and dating in the modern age.

Gavin and Stacey – So funny and uplifting. Rewatched every episode and couldn't stop smiling, even with a chemotherapy pump in my arm.

Roland Garros and Wimbledon – I'm a tennis tragic from way back. The French Open got me through some tough days during treatment and Ash Barty's Wimbledon victory filled my heart.

Would I Lie To You? – The irresistible trio of Lee Mack, David Mitchell and Rob Bryden.

Grand Designs – Building and interior inspiration, invariably over time and budget.

MasterChef – 2021 was the best of this (Australian) series in ages, despite the ads.

The Voice – As above, hate the ads but loved the positive vibe this year. Just what I needed.

Have You Been Paying Attention? – Ditto re ads but very funny show with Sam Pang et al.

> *The best entertainment speaks to the human condition in an honest way.* ~ Gregory Hines

Films

I have eclectic taste and will watch pretty much any good film from any genre except horror. I'm a sucker for a good romcom, anything by Richard Curtis, anything with Emma Thompson, period dramas and tearjerkers like The Notebook. Here is a minuscule sample of films I've discovered or revisited on streaming services this year:

Emma – The latest version with Anya Taylor Joy from the Queen's Gambit.

Hamilton – The film of the stage musical. Can't wait to see it in the theatre.

Little Women – Latest version.

Viceroy's House – Had never seen this before.

Bend it Like Beckham – An oldie but a goodie.

The Man Who Knew Infinity – Love, love, love Dev Patel.

The African Doctor – A gentle French film.

The Climb – Loosely based on the book by the first Senegalese man to climb Everest.

The Railway Man – Colin Firth finds redemption in this harrowing tale.

… and lots of random romantic dramas and comedies on the many (far too many) streaming services we have.

Three films I avoided (for obvious reasons): *Beaches*, *The Fault in Our Stars*, *Terms of Endearment*.

Everything I learned I learned from the movies. ~ Audrey Hepburn

Books

I'm a huge reader, as if you couldn't guess. And my reading material is as eclectic as my playlists. Here are just some of the books I've read or revisited this past year:

Phosphorescence, by Julia Baird – This beautiful book really did fill me up with light.

The Daily Stoic: 366 Meditations on Wisdom, Perseverance and *The Art of Living* by Ryan Holiday and Stephen Hanselman – Packed full of wise words and insight.

Untamed, by Glennon Doyle – A call to stop being who you think you should be and become who you are. I'm working on it, Glennon!

The Gifts of Imperfection, by Brené Brown – Lots that resonated here. I'm trying hard to find my awkward, brave and kind best self!

The Thursday Murder Club, by Richard Osman – Such fun. A total release.

Grown Ups, by Marian Keyes – I love MK. I have no idea how she juggled all the characters in this book. Impressive.

The Mistake, by Katie McMahon – Stumbled across this on my Kindle and really enjoyed it.

Messy, Wonderful Us, by Catherine Isaac – Another Kindle special. Quality chick lit.

Moonflower Murders, by Anthony Horowitz – Really enjoyed the interplay of fact and fiction here.

The Wife and the Widow, by Christian White – a masterfully twisty and original thriller.

The Holiday, by T M Logan – Beware holidays with friends. You might not all come home.

Let me Lie, by Clare Mackintosh – Another twisty thriller par excellence. I'd love to be able to plot like this.

The Safe Place, by Anna Downes – A psychological thriller set in the south of France. My French nannying days were not quite so eventful.

Playing Nice, by J P Delaney – Can't really remember this one but I know I enjoyed it.

Never Greener, by Ruth Jones – First novel by the co-writer of Gavin and Stacey. How talented can one woman be?

The Godmothers, by Monica McInerney – Another winner. Easy to read, well written and hugely enjoyable.

… and many, many more.

We read to know we're not alone. ~ William Nicholson

Books are the quietest and most constant of friends; they are the most accessible and wisest of counsellors and the most patient of teachers.
~ Charles William Eliot

Walking

When I was battling depression, I started walking regularly and I haven't really stopped since. I try to walk for at least an hour each day. When I was diagnosed with cancer, just keep walking became one of my mantras. In 2014, I walked part of the Camino de Santiago and hope to return one day to walk the rest. In the time of COVID and the year of Alan, these were some of my favourite paths and tracks:

In and around City Beach, Floreat, Swanbourne, Scarborough and Trigg, on coastal paths or barefoot on the beach.

Take me to the lakes (great song Tay Tay) – Perry Lakes; Jackadder Lake; Herdsman Lake; Lake Claremont.

Trigg Bushland.

The coastal track from Dunsborough to the Cape Naturaliste Lighthouse.

Anywhere along the Cape-to-Cape track in South-West WA,

The Nullaki side of Ocean Beach, Denmark.

All truly great thoughts are conceived while walking.
~ Friedrich Nietzsche

Walking is man's (and woman's) best medicine. ~ Hippocrates

Random tips and advice

I have learnt that, as with depression, there is no one size fits all with cancer. You have to do it your way. Here are some things that helped me and may be useful to others:

Stay away from Dr Google.

Use social media carefully. While it's great to connect with friends and support groups and receive lots of virtual love and hugs, rabbit holes of misinformation are to be avoided.

Cancer is a bit like childbirth and parenthood; everyone has an opinion. Always remember that it's your body, your illness, your treatment – your choice.

The bone-crushing tiredness caused by treatment is like nothing else. Sometimes you can't fight it and all you can do is surrender.

Take advantage of cancer support therapies available if they appeal, such as massage, reflexology, Reiki and counselling. I did a few things at the beginning of my treatment but in the end developed appointment fatigue and preferred to go my own way. Don't feel you have to do everything on offer. Whatever you choose or don't choose to do is just fine.

I hit a wall during treatment when I thought I couldn't go on, but by telling myself "this too shall pass" and drawing on something deep within me, something I don't really understand, I somehow kept going.

Dealing with friends and family can be tricky. Try not to worry or feel guilty about offending people (easier said than done). If they don't understand why you don't feel like talking, why you don't immediately reply to messages, why you don't always want their advice, however well-meaning, why you need to hide away, then that's their problem. It's not about them, it's about what you need and your recovery.

Sometimes you find support or a new friendship when you least expect it. Embrace it all and be thankful.

Beware the positivity police: No one can be positive all the time, and the expectation to be so can be draining.

Listen to your body and do what you need to do on any given day. If that means staying in bed, then get a big pile of books and magazines and do it. I lived in pyjamas and trackie pants for weeks.

Keep up a gentle exercise regime – check with your medical team first, of course.

Get outside, at least once a day, whatever the weather. Preferably barefoot.

Embrace stillness and silence. Tune into nature. Listen to birdsong, the ocean, the rain. Feel the wind on your face.

Practise gratitude, seek out joy. However bad I felt, I tried to find something to be grateful for and one little pocket of joy each day.

Get creative. Having cancer gave me more time to write, listen to music, take photographs, cook and play the piano.

Photography is a way of feeling, of touching, of loving ... it remembers little things, long after you have forgotten everything. ~ Aaron Siskind

Tears are words that need to be written. ~ Paulo Coelho

A few useful websites

beyondblue.org.au

cancerwa.asn.au

cancer.org.au

solariscancercare.org.au

community.macmillan.org.uk

chat10looks3.com

thriveglobal.com

brenebrown.com

Extreme darkness rekindles the radiant flame of the human spirit. You are much stronger than you think. ~ Anthon St. Maarten

Author's note

A few years ago, I wrote and walked my way out of a period of depression and anxiety so debilitating I almost didn't survive. I thought I'd had my mid-life crisis. Turns out there was another curveball heading my way.

This time though, it was different. When I was depressed, I didn't want to be alive. When I found out I had cancer, life seemed like the most precious gift.

In the days after my diagnosis, I somehow managed to keep walking every day. *Just keep walking* became my mantra. I'd put on my headphones, crank up the volume and hope it would all just disappear.

And I wrote. When I need to be on my own and shut out the world, I always have writing. I write what I cannot say. It is so very cathartic. While preparing for my first trip to hospital I packed my laptop as an afterthought and started typing in the admissions' waiting room.

My first book, *Changing Lightbulbs*, was written when I'd come through the worst of my depression and was well on the way to recovery. This time, the story unfolded as it happened and I had no idea how it would end.

Sharing my cancer diagnosis was tough. I know vulnerability is strength and all that, but it's damn hard. I wondered who would want to read a memoir about cancer. Then a friend told me it could help others, just as writing and speaking about depression and anxiety resonated with so many people, and I knew I had to share my story.

I hope this book will help you support a friend or family member facing their own challenges, or inspire you to raise much needed funds for cancer research. And if you are going through a tough time, I hope it brings some comfort and helps you feel less alone. We are never alone.

There is nothing quite like a cancer diagnosis to make you see the importance of taking each day as it comes. Of living in the moment. Of avoiding people who deplete you. Of channelling what little energy you have into the things that matter. Of delighting in fleeting moments of happiness and finding joy amidst the pain.

I would never presume to tell anyone how to live their life: three ways to do this, five ways to do that. It's not my style. And while I may have inadvertently offered some advice, this is most certainly not a self-help book. I will say this, though. Never ignore that nagging feeling that tells you something isn't right in your body.

Acknowledgements

All the people in this book are real, but some names have been changed to protect privacy.

Deepest thanks go to my friends, both near and far, for their unconditional love, support and kindness.

To all the medical staff I encountered along this journey, and those behind the scenes, the consultants and surgeons and anaesthetists and pathologists and nurses and radiologists and all the ancillary workers who make this world a better place by showing up each day so that we can be healed, thank you, thank you, thank you.

Thank you to Rhianna King for reading the first draft of this book, for the invaluable feedback and for believing in my writing.

Thank you to Ian for always walking by my side, especially when the going gets tough, and for his unwavering confidence in me.

Finally, thank you to Daniel and Ben for inspiring me to be a better person and for lighting up my life with all the chats and songs and love and laughter.

SUE TREDGET

About the author

Sue Tredget grew up in Northern Ireland and studied Modern Languages at Leeds University. She lived and worked in France, Spain and England before moving to Perth, Western Australia in 1999.

In 2014, Sue took a break from teaching to write and travel. She stayed at a retreat in India, travelled solo around Italy and walked part of the Camino de Santiago, among other adventures.

Sue now teaches part-time and writes whenever she can. She is also the author of *Changing Lightbulbs: A journey through anxiety and depression*, *Transformation: A collection of poems to heal and replenish the spirit*, and the children's picture book series *My Colour Collection*.

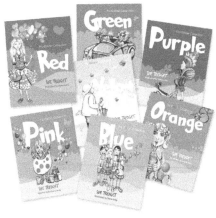

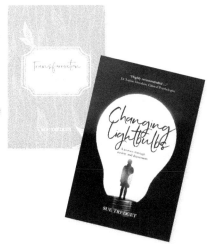

www.suetredget.com

www.facebook.com@suetredgetauthor
www.instagram.com@suetredgetauthor

SUE TREDGET

SUE TREDGET

Milton Keynes UK
Ingram Content Group UK Ltd.
UKHW020731131123
432471UK00004B/45